FLUORIDES AND
DENTAL CARIES

FLUORIDES AND DENTAL CARIES

Contemporary Concepts for Practitioners and Students

Edited by

ERNEST NEWBRUN, D.M.D., Ph.D.

Professor of Oral Biology
Chairman, Section Biological Sciences
* School of Dentistry*
University of California, San Francisco

With a Foreword by
Yngve Ericsson

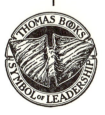

CHARLES C THOMAS • PUBLISHER
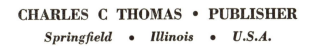
Springfield • *Illinois* • *U.S.A.*

Published and Distributed Throughout the World by
CHARLES C THOMAS • PUBLISHER
BANNERSTONE HOUSE
301–327 East Lawrence Avenue, Springfield, Illinois, U.S.A.
NATCHEZ PLANTATION HOUSE

© *1972, by* CHARLES C THOMAS • PUBLISHER
ISBN 0-398-02563-0
Library of Congress Catalog Card Number: 72-79195

Printed in the United States of America
CC-11

It is not the function of a university to cram the heads of students with as many facts as can be squeezed in. Its proper task is to lead them into habits of critical examination and an understanding of canons and criteria which bear on all subject matters.

BERTRAND RUSSELL

CONTRIBUTORS

STANLEY B. HEIFETZ, B.A., D.D.S., M.P.H.
Community Programs Section
Caries Prevention and Research Branch
National Institute of Dental Research
Bethesda, Maryland

HAROLD C. HODGE, Ph.D.
Professor of Pharmacology and Oral Biology
University of California
San Francisco, California

HERSCHEL S. HOROWITZ, D.D.S., M.P.H.
Chief, Community Programs Section
Caries Prevention and Research Branch
National Institute of Dental Research
Bethesda, Maryland

HOWARD M. MYERS, D.D.S., M.S., Ph.D., M.A.
Professor and Chairman, Department of Biochemistry
School of Dentistry, University of the Pacific
San Francisco, California

STEVEN J. SILVERSTEIN, D.M.D., M.P.H.
Lecturer in Preventive Dentistry and Community Health
School of Dentistry, University of California
San Francisco, California

SAMUEL J. WYCOFF, B.S., D.M.D., M.P.H.
Associate Professor in Residence
Chairman of Division of Preventive Dentistry and Community Health
University of California
San Francisco, California

ISADORE ZIPKIN, A.B., M.S., Ph.D.
Professor of Periodontology
School of Dentistry, University of California
San Francisco, California

FOREWORD

I AM HONORED to have been asked by the Editor to write a short foreword to this book. At first I thought this request came because my work for the World Health Organization might qualify me to comment on international aspects of its content, but the Editor himself has firsthand experience from three continents. Nor would my scientific contributions to the oral and general biology of fluorides indicate superior judgement when the authors of the individual chapters are all top-ranking scientists of international repute. However, my humble experience as author and editor of textbooks enables me to appreciate particularly the creation of this book on fluorides and dental caries, for I am aware of the need in this field for information in textbook form and of the difficulty of meeting this need.

At a time when diffuse fears of chemicals, poisons, and environmental pollution have become widespread among the public, it is imperative that both dentists and dental hygienists are well informed on the properties of fluorides and their proper uses and advantages as agents for prevention of dental caries. This is valid both for clinical use of these agents by the profession and for answering adequately the numerous enquiries by patients, to whom explanations should be given at the level of knowledge of the individual. The professional man or woman should never feel inhibited by lack of basic knowledge from participating in community debates on such matters as water fluoridation and collective fluoride applications in schools.

Adequate knowledge in this field is not easily compiled from handbooks, monographs, and scientific and professional journals, and it is therefore gratifying that a textbook of this type, scope, and quality has been compiled and is available to students and practitioners. The scientific competence

ix

and experience of all the contributors to the book guarantee
standards of basic knowledge, current interest, and reliabil-
ity in the contents which are outstanding, even for the home-
land of fluoridation.

YNGVE ERICSSON

PREFACE

Today's dentist is expected to be an expert on many aspects of fluorides, by his patients and the community. This is not a simple task. There is a vast literature on this topic, and the dentist is often faced with the problem of having to obtain his information from a variety of sources, e.g. textbooks on public health dentistry, pedodontics, pharmacology, sociology, as well as a variety of special monographs and articles in dental journals. Accordingly, this is an attempt to bring together the information currently available on fluoride as a caries-preventive agent. This book will provide the material in a readily accessible form. Its purpose is also to stimulate interest to read further.

Fluorides and Dental Caries has been prepared primarily for the teaching of undergraduate dental students and dental hygienists. It is also intended for use by graduate students in oral biology, pedodontics and public health.

It is recommended that the class be divided into groups of no more than 15 to 20 students to participate in seminar discussions on the various areas within this topic. Students should be familiar with the subject matter for the week so that they can actively participate in order to gain the most from the class discussion. To facilitate reading, detailed references have not always been included in the text; however, major review articles and monographs are listed at the end of each section.

The authors of each chapter have expertise in the research and/or teaching of fluoride as a caries-preventive agent. Chapter 2, "Fluoride Dentifrices," has been adapted from a review on therapeutic dentifrices which appeared in the *Journal of Public Health Dentistry, 30*:206-211, 1970. Chapter 3, "Current Status of Topical Fluorides in Preventive Dentistry," was originally published as a report by the Council of Dental Therapeutics in the *Journal of the American Dental Association, 81*:166-177, 1970. The major part of Chapter 7, "Fluoride Toxicology," is reprinted from the *Journal of Occupational Medicine, 10*:273-277, 1968.

The editor appreciates the willing cooperation of his colleagues in the preparation of this book.

ERNEST NEWBRUN

CONTENTS

FLUORIDES AND
DENTAL CARIES

Chapter 1

WATER FLUORIDATION AND DIETARY FLUORIDE

ERNEST NEWBRUN

WATER FLUORIDATION

Dental Fluorosis

As EARLY AS the nineteenth century calcified tissues were know to contain fluoride. Magitot in France and Crichton-Browne in England speculated that fluoride might fortify tooth structure. However, the earliest epidemiological studies were concerned with the disfiguring effects on enamel observed in certain locations in Italy, Iceland, Argentina, North Africa and the southwestern parts of the United States. In 1901, enamel defects and black teeth were reported among the inhabitants of towns near Naples. The etiology was connected with volcanic fumes contaminating the drinking water. The following year, brown staining of teeth was recorded in El Paso County, Colorado. In 1916, a dentist, Frederick McKay, practicing in Colorado noticed staining of the teeth of many of his patients. He invited Dr. G. V. Black to join him in a local survey which attracted national publicity. At that time this condition was associated with the communal water supply, often from deep wells, but the etiological agent was unknown. The name "Colorado brown stain" was replaced by the term "mottling," as the condition was recognized in other communities in Arizona, New Mexico and Texas as well as Colorado. It is now called endemic dental fluorosis. Several degrees of fluorosis have been recognized and given a numerical value for epidemiological scoring (Table I).

An individual with two or more teeth in a higher grade is placed in that category. In its mildest form fluorosis is not a disfigurement. Tooth discoloration, mottling and

TABLE I

CLASSIFICATION OF DEGREE OF FLUOROSIS

Grade of Fluorosis	Description of Fluorosis	DFI Score
Normal	None	0
Questionable	A few white flecks or white spots	0.5
Very Mild	Small opaque, paper-white areas involving less than 25% of the surface	1.0
Mild	White opacities are more extensive but do not involve more than 50% of the surface	2.0
Moderate	Distinct brown stain, all enamel surfaces affected	3.0
Severe	Besides brown staining, the tooth is worn and hypoplastic. All enamel surfaces affected	4.0

enamel hypoplasia may arise from other causes besides fluoride. For this reason the specific term "dental fluorosis" is more appropriate when fluoride is known to be the causative agent. In the differential diagnosis of dental fluorosis it must be distinguished from idiopathic white flecks of enamel, iatrogenic discoloration from tetracyclines and hypoplasia resulting from exanthematous fevers. More rarely, endogenous discoloration of the teeth may be a result of hereditary dentinogenesis imperfecta or erythroblastosis fetalis (Rh incompatibility). Exogenous stains produced by tobacco, and pellicle can readily be differentiated from dental fluorosis.

In 1925, concern because of dental discoloration prompted the inhabitants of Oakley, Idaho, to switch from deep artesian wells (1000 to 2500 ft) to a shallow water supply. Although this did not alter the staining of teeth already calcified, in subsequent years no new fluorosis developed. The initial discovery in 1931 that high levels of fluoride in the water supply caused the enamel discoloration came as a result of advances in the chemical analysis of fluoride. Samples of drinking water from Bauxite, Arkansas, a town with a high incidence of enamel disfiguration, were assayed by H. V. Churchill, who found 13.7 parts per million (ppm) of fluoride. Water samples from other locations showing endemic fluorosis were also found to have elevated fluoride levels by Smith, Lantz and Smith in Arizona and Velu in France. The specific addition of fluoride to the diet of experimental animals was shown to produce dental fluorosis proportional to the concentration in the diet. Exactly how fluorides produce enamel defects is not known at the molecular level. Ameloblasts appear to be more sensitive to fluoride than are other cells in the body. The deciduous teeth are rarely affected and only at high levels of fluoride intake. Fluorosed enamel (i.e. from areas > 2.0 ppm), in addition to showing a higher degree of pigmentation, is more permeable to dyes, more radiolucent and has a lower surface hardness. These alterations are doubtlessly manifestations of the altered function of the ameloblasts during enamel formation. The mechanism whereby fluorides reduce caries will be discussed in a later chapter.

Dental Caries and Fluoride

It had been noticed that fluorosed teeth, though sometimes hypoplastic, appeared less caries prone. Extensive epidemiological surveys of dental caries prevalence and dental fluorosis of communities in the U.S.A. were carried out by H. Trendley Dean and others working for the United States Public Health Service during the late 1930s. They examined 7,257 children 12 to 14 years old in 21 cities of four different states with a natural high or low fluoride content in the public water supply (Fig. 1).

Number of cities studied	Number of children examined	Number of DMF teeth per 100 examinees	Fluoride content of water (ppm)
11	3 867		< 0.5
3	1 140		0.5 - 0.9
4	1 403		1.0 - 1.4
3	847		> 1.4

Figure 1. Data from 21 cities grouped according to fluoride content of drinking water.

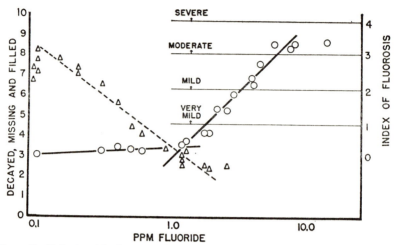

Figure 2. Relationship between fluoride content of the drinking water, caries prevalence and dental fluorosis. DMF – – – – – DFI——————— (Courtesy Drs. Hodge and Smith [1954] Fluoridation as a Public Health Measure, [AAAS.])

Clearly there was an inverse relationship between caries prevalence and fluoride concentration in the drinking water. On the other hand there was a direct relationship between the dental fluorosis index (DFI) and the concentration of fluoride in the drinking water (Fig. 2).

At a concentration of 1.0 to 1.2 ppm of fluoride, the risk of dental fluorosis is minimal and not appreciably greater than at much lower levels of fluoride. However, there is a significant protection against caries compared to communities with less than 0.5 ppm of fluoride.

It has since been documented that the effect of fluoride protection is not limited to young children. Adults who have continually consumed fluoridated waters have lower tooth mortality and lower DMFT scores than the corresponding age group living in a low fluoride area (Fig. 3). At each age level the DMFT score is approximately 60 percent lower in the community drinking fluoride-containing water.

Although the overall caries reduction is about 60 per-

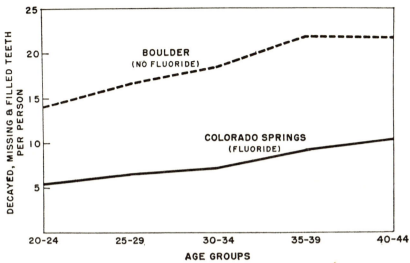

Figure 3. Caries in adults living in a fluoride and low-fluoride area. Boulder: Trace—0.1 ppm fluoride. Colorado Springs: 2.5 ppm fluoride.

cent, a careful examination of the data indicates a selective protection of the proximal and buccolingual surfaces in comparison to the occlusal surfaces. For example, the caries-inhibitory effect of fluoride on proximal surfaces of upper incisors is 85 to 95 percent, on smooth surfaces of molars 50 to 60 percent, but only about 20 to 25 percent for pit and fissure lesions.

Fluoride Supplementation of Water Supplies

North American Clinical Trials

After establishing the threshold of concentration of fluoride in natural water supplies at which objectionable fluorosis occurs and the concentration of fluoride which provides significant protection, the next step was to find out if fluoride added to the domestic water supply could reduce caries prevalence. In 1945 to 1947 four independent clinical studies were undertaken at Grand Rapids, Michigan, Newburgh, New York, Evanston, Illinois, and Brantford, Ontario. At each of these cities fluoride was supplemented in the communal water supply to approximately 1.0 ppm. Neighboring cities having similar characteristics but with low fluoride levels were used as controls. After 15 years of water fluoridation, children ages 12 to 14 years born and residing in the trial cities had 50 to 70 percent lower DMFT scores (Table II) than children in the control cities or children in the same community prior to fluoridation.

Very thorough medical examinations of the children accompanied both Newburgh-Kingston and Grand Rapids-Muskegon fluoridation studies. No significant differences were found in the health or growth and development between children in study and control cities. The Newburgh examination was very detailed and included tonsillectomy rates, height and weight, onset of menstruation, bone density by x-rays of hands and knees, skeletal maturation, hemoglobin level, erythrocyte count, leukocyte count, skin-moisture, texture, color, eruptions, and urinalysis. The conclusion of this long-term pediatric study was that there was no indication of any systemic effects, adverse or otherwise, except for the reduction in caries, from the use of fluoridated water.

International Progress Toward Water Fluoridation

The success of these initial trials in the U.S.A. and Canada was so convincing that further water fluoridation programs were started in other communities in the U.S.A. and elsewhere. In several countries, specially appointed

TABLE II

COMPARISON OF CARIES SCORES IN FLUORIDE-SUPPLEMENTED AND LOW-FLUORIDE AREAS

City	Fluoride Status	Year	Age	DMFT/ child	% Difference
Grand Rapids	(No F)	1945	12–14 yrs	9.5	—55.5
	(F)	1959		4.26	
Evanston	(No F)	1946	12–14 yrs	9.03	—48.8
	(F)	1959		4.66	
Sarnia	(No F)	1959	12–14 yrs	7.46	—56.7
Brantford	(F)	1959		3.23	
Kingston	(No F)	1960	13–14 yrs	12.46	—70.1
Newburgh	(F)	1960		3.73	

commissions and other bodies have recommended water fluoridation as a public health measure.

In the United Kingdom, reductions in caries experience have been reported following fluoridation of the drinking water in communities in Sutton (England), Kilmarnoch (Scotland) and Anglesey (Wales). After almost 16 years of fluoridation at Tiel (Netherlands) there has not only been a decrease in the caries prevalence but also a 90 percent reduction in the mean number of extractions per child. In the U.S.S.R. results at Norilsk after seven years of water fluoridation show a 43 percent reduction in dental caries among seven-year-olds and a 33 percent decrease among eight-year-olds. The effectiveness of water fluoridation has also been demonstrated by trials in the Southern Hemisphere in Hastings and Lower Hutt (New Zealand) and Tamworth and Yass (Australia).

Owing to a lack of standardization in reporting, statistics on reduction in prevalence and incidence of dental caries after fluoridation are difficult to compare and summarize in a uniform manner. Numerous studies have been conducted among different age groups, but for varying lengths of time and using a variety of methods for examination. Nevertheless, the finding of substantial reductions in dental caries following fluoridation of the water supplies has now been reproduced in many different communities in the U.S.A. and throughout the world. The consistency of these findings among populations living under diverse environmental and cultural conditions is most impressive.

The available information concerning international adoption of water fluoridation programs is summarized in Table III. Progress has been slow in both eastern and western Europe, with the exception of Ireland and the Netherlands. North America, Australia, New Zealand and some countries in South America have the most fluoridation programs underway.

At the end of 1971 over 95 million United States residents (59 percent of the population on public water supplies)

TABLE III

WORLD WIDE WATER FLUORIDATION *

County or Territory	Year First Project Started	Population Served by Fluoride-Supplemented Water	Percentage of Total Population Served with Fluoridated Water †
Australia	1956	5,000,000	41
Belgium	1956	400,000	4
Brazil	1953	2,930,000	3.1
Canada	1945	7,300,000	34
Chile	1953	3,300,000	39
Colombia	1953	2,520,000	12
Czechoslovakia	1958	1,000,000	10
El Salvador	1956	1,380,000	50
Federal Republic of Germany	1952	6,000	0.01
Finland	1959	60,000	1.3
Hong Kong	1961	3,570,000	100
Ireland	1964	1,350,000	47
Japan	1952	....	....
Kuwait	1968	676,000	100
Malaysia	....	3,000,000	25
Mexico	1960	1,750,000	4.4
Netherlands	1953	3,000,000	20
New Zealand	1953	1,205,000	43
Panama	1950	560,000	40
Papua and New Guinea	1966	38,000	1.7
Paraguay	1959	220,000	9
Poland	1967	500,000	5
Puerto Rico	1953	1,820,000	67
Rumania	....	100,000	0.5
Ryukyu Islands	....	740,000	78
Sarawak	....	180,000	....
Singapore	1958	2,000,000	100
Sweden	1952	130,000 (discontinued)	....
Switzerland	1960	274,000	5
United Kingdom	1955	2,305,000	4
USA	1945	86,000,000	40
USSR	1960	13,000,000	4
Venezuela	1952	70,000	1

* Based on information supplied by governments, the International Dental Federation, WHO Chronicle, European Public Health Committee, Council of Europe and Dental Section Department of Health Services, Pan American Sanitary Bureau of the WHO.

† The percentage of total population served with fluoridated water refers only to those receiving controlled fluoridated water. Calculation of the percentage of population served by communal water supplies receiving controlled or natural fluoride containing water gives considerably higher values for some countries.

were drinking fluoridated water (see Figs. 4 and 5). Of these, 86 million were served by fluoride-supplemented supply systems. In California, however, only 18 percent of the state's population are enjoying the benefits of this preventive measure (see Table IV). Accordingly, California ranks forty-third out of the 50 states as far as progress towards communal water fluoridation is concerned. In contrast, in states like Colorado, Connecticut, Illinois, Maryland and Rhode Island over 70 percent of the total population are served with fluoridated water.

School Water Fluoridation

Because central water supplies are not available to large segments of the world's population, other methods of caries prevention have been sought. Schools that have no central water systems usually have private wells which can readily be fluoridated. Initial studies have used 2.5 to 5 ppm fluoride in the schools in an attempt to approximate the total fluoride intake of children who drink optimally fluoridated water on a full-time basis. No objectionable dental fluorosis has resulted. After 12 years of school fluoridation, children at a rural school had a 39 percent reduction in dental caries compared to prefluoridation figures and a 65 percent reduction in the rate of extraction between 1958 and 1970. Additional studies are indicated to develop maximum effectiveness of this procedure.

Effect of Stopping Water Fluoridation

Most studies on the effectiveness of fluoridation have been based on communities where there has been a continuous presence of fluoride in the water supply once fluoridation had begun. It might be questioned whether the effect of water fluoridation lasts beyond the period of utilization or whether, as in the bony skeleton, withdrawal of fluoride from the water supply results in loss of fluoride (and its protective effect) from the enamel surface. Fortunately, there are only a few communities where this has been the case and then only for a few years. As the caries rates increased these communities became sufficiently concerned to reinstitute fluoridation. One such example is

TABLE IV
PERCENT OF POPULATION SERVED WITH NATURAL & CONTROLLED FLUORIDATED WATER *
DECEMBER 31, 1971

	Percentage of Population on Public Water Supplies Served with Fluoridated Water	Percentage of Total Population Served with Fluoridated Water
United States	58.7	45.5
Alabama	40.6	25.6
Alaska	79.9	44.0
Arizona	19.6	17.3
Arkansas	67.7	36.7
California	19.4	18.2
Colorado	89.5	73.3
Connecticut	90.6	72.6
Delaware	54.3	40.2
Dist. of Columbia	100.0	100.0
Florida	37.4	28.9
Georgia	68.0	47.3
Hawaii	13.2	12.8
Idaho	27.2	17.7
Illinois	98.1	84.4
Indiana	88.9	58.6
Iowa	80.7	55.0
Kansas	58.8	44.8
Kentucky	81.0	46.1
Louisiana	10.4	7.9
Maine	58.9	35.1
Maryland	98.1	76.9
Massachusetts	13.3	12.4
Michigan	90.7	63.6
Minnesota	98.0	73.0
Mississippi	43.6	21.9
Missouri	61.7	45.2
Montana	28.9	19.3
Nebraska	67.2	47.9
Nevada	3.8	3.3
New Hampshire	17.7	11.5
New Jersey	14.8	13.0
New Mexico	53.4	38.9
New York	75.8	66.3
North Carolina	74.9	37.9
North Dakota	91.5	48.0
Ohio	53.5	42.0
Oklahoma	74.9	56.4
Oregon	21.8	16.4
Pennsylvania	52.4	42.0
Rhode Island	90.1	80.7
South Carolina	64.3	36.1
South Dakota	90.6	52.9
Tennessee	67.5	43.9
Texas	63.3	50.8
Utah	2.7	2.5
Vermont	45.8	26.5
Virginia	95.5	61.8
Washington	46.4	38.4
West Virginia	83.0	50.9
Wisconsin	94.8	61.4
Wyoming	40.1	29.7
Puerto Rico	92.4	66.7

* U.S. Dept. of Health, Education and Welfare, NIH, April 1972.

Antigo, Wisconsin, where fluoridation began in 1949, was discontinued in November 1960, and resumed in October 1965. The dental caries experience of kindergarten children in Antigo is shown in Table V.

The available data show that the caries-protective effect is diminished when fluoride intake is discontinued. Careful study of caries increments of the older children who had already ingested fluoride during some period of tooth formation indicates that the maximum inhibitory effect of fluoride is not permanent, but tends slowly to be lost. Maximum caries inhibition requires continuous exposure of the enamel surface to fluoridated waters. These findings suggest that water fluoridation acts not only by supplying this trace element systemically but also locally to plaque and the enamel surface.

Optimum Levels of Fluoride

It is important to realize that there is no single optimum level which is valid at all times and for all places. Several factors must be taken into consideration in order to establish the desirable water concentration for a particular community.

The optimal concentration of fluoride in the water depends upon the annual average of maximum daily air temperatures in the community, as this influences the amount of water ingested. Recommended concentrations according to Public Health Service Drinking Water Standards 1962 are shown in Table VI. Some communities may also adjust the fluoride concentration to allow for seasonal variations in temperature.

TABLE V

DENTAL CARIES EXPERIENCE RELATED TO STOPPING
WATER FLUORIDATION

Year	Number of Children Examined	Mean def.	% Increase from 1960
1960	125	2.5	....
1964	131	4.8	92
1966	103	5.3	112

TABLE VI

RELATIONSHIP OF OPTIMAL LEVEL OF FLUORIDE TO TEMPERATURE

Annual Average of Maximum Daily Air Temperature		Recommended Control Limits Fluoride (mg/liter)		
°C	°F	Lower	Optimum	Upper
10.0–12.1	50.0–53.7	0.9	1.2	1.7
12.2–14.6	53.8–58.3	0.8	1.1	1.5
14.7–17.7	58.4–63.8	0.8	1.0	1.3
17.8–21.4	63.9–70.6	0.7	0.9	1.2
21.5–26.2	70.7–79.2	0.7	0.8	1.0
26.3–32.5	79.3–90.5	0.6	0.7	0.8

Controlled fluoridation is defined as the conscious maintenance of the optimal fluoride concentration in the water supply. Several different fluorine compounds can be used, provided they will dissociate to supply the necessary fluoride ion. The compounds currently in use include sodium fluoride, sodium silicofluoride, fluosilicic acid, ammonium fluosilicate and calcium fluoride. They are added by automatic feeding machinery in either solution or dry form. The machinery may operate to deliver either a measured volume or a measured dry weight of the compound within a given time interval. In addition, regular monitoring of the fluoride concentration is carried out by colorimetric assay or continuous measurement of electroconductivity.

DIETARY FLUORIDE

Fluoridation of drinking water is not universally feasible because many areas, especially rural areas, are not served by communal water supplies. In order to extend the dental benefits of fluoride to persons residing in these areas, dietary alternatives providing a continual fluoride intake have been explored. Different vehicles have been proposed and to some extent tested; these include salt, milk, flour and fluoride tablets or solutions.

The daily water consumption for an average adult is in the range of 1 to 1.5 liters, which if it contains optimal levels of fluoride provides 1.0 to 1.5 mg fluoride per day. Accordingly, this is the level aimed at when supplementing by dietary means. It should be recognized that the total amount of fluoride ingested is greater than this and has been estimated to be a minimum of 3.2 mg/day, the additional fluoride coming from the regular diet. Most foods contain about 0.5 mg fluoride per kg, however certain foods contain relatively higher concentrations of fluoride, such as fish, tea and some wines.

Fluoride Ingestion with Salt

The addition of fluoride to table salt has been practiced in some parts of Switzerland for several years. The World Health Organization recently initiated a fluoridated salt study in Colombia, South America. There is a precedent for this route of supplementation in that iodized salt has been found beneficial against goitre. The kitchen salt is sprayed with sodium fluoride to contain 200 mg NaF per kg. Based on average salt consumption ($\cong$ 4 gm/adult/day), this represents a supplementation of only about 0.4 mg fluoride/adult/day or about a third of the desired level. In spite of this low dosage, a 22 percent reduction in DMFT scores after 4.5 years of unsupervised use was found in eight- to 9-year-old children. This method has an inherent disadvantage in that it is difficult to accommodate to varying but suboptimal levels of natural fluoride in the water supplies.

Fluoride Ingestion with Milk

Few studies have tested milk as a vehicle for fluoride supplementation, and these have involved only small groups of children. The published results indicate a positive caries-preventive effect, however much more clinical evidence is needed before establishing this route as a satisfactory one. In fact, milk has certain disadvantages. Water, bread and salt consumption during childhood increases fairly regularly with increasing age. Milk, on the other hand, is ingested in relatively large amounts during the first two years but then consumption decreases. Furthermore, the addition of fluoride to milk in a fairly large number of dairies might create some technical difficulties. It it also difficult to separate distribution of such milk between closely approximating fluoride and nonfluoride areas. The great variability and irregularity of milk consumption habits in different geographical regions, seasons of the year and age groups are serious problems.

Fluoride Tablets or Drops

Fluoride can be administered to children as a daily supplement in tablet or liquid form. It is important that the supplement be taken on a regular basis over prolonged periods of time, particularly during the period of tooth calcification, if any substantial benefit is to be expected. This requires careful supervision and strong motivation on the part of the parent. To avoid the risk of possible misuse or ineffective use, The Council on Dental Therapeutics of the American Dental Association "strongly advises against the indiscriminate distribution or casual prescription of supplements of dietary fluoride." It also recommends that no more than 264 mg of NaF be dispensed at any one time and that each package be labelled: Caution—Store out of reach of children. Generic prescriptions can be used, and there are also several proprietary sodium fluoride preparations. There is no rationale for combining fluoride with vitamin preparations and their use is not acceptable. The dosage of fluoride can not be treated as lightly as vitamin dosage.

The following is a sample prescription for a child of three years or older:

Ṛ Sodium fluoride tablets 2.2 mg
Dispense 100
Sig. One tablet each day in ½ glass of water or juice
Caution: Store out of reach of children

For infants under two years old, dissolve one tablet to a quart of water which can be used in the preparation of formulas and other foods. Children two or three years old should take ½ tablet (1.1 mg) each day.

The above prescription and dosage apply to areas where there is no substantial fluoride in the drinking water. In areas where there is some but insufficient fluoride, the Council suggests the following (Table VII) be used as a guide.

In such locations, a fluoride solution is preferable as it permits a better control of the dosage. The following prescription can be used:

> ℞ Sodium fluoride 0.26 gm
> Distilled water, to make 60 ml
> Dispense in plastic dropper bottle
> that delivers 20 drops per each ml
> Sig. Use .... drops each day in ½ glass water or juice

Each drop of this solution contains 0.1 mg fluoride ion. The appropriate number of drops should be specified on the label based on the adjusted allowances shown in Table VII and the age of the child.

Communities with natural fluoride in the water in the amount of 0.7 ppm or more are listed in a U.S.P.H.S. publication *Natural Fluoride Content of Community Water Supplies 1969* and communities using controlled fluoridated water in another U.S.P.H.S. publication *Fluoridation Census 1969* (see Figs. 4 and 5). If your community does not fall in either of these two categories, fluoride supplementation is indicated for cooperative and motivated patients. Information as to the fluoride concentration in your area can be obtained from the local municipal water supplier.

The effectiveness of fluoride tablets in reducing caries in children has been documented in several studies. When

TABLE VII

RECOMMENDED DIETARY FLUORIDE SUPPLEMENTATION

WATER FLUORIDE	ADJUSTED ADULT ALLOWANCE	
ppm	*Sodium fluoride mg per day*	*Provides fluoride ion mg per day*
0.0	2.2	1.0
0.2	1.8	0.8
0.4	1.3	0.6
0.6	0.9	0.4

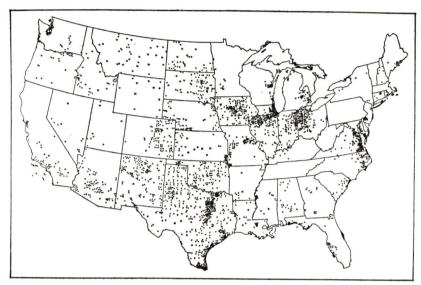

Figure 4. Distribution of communities with 0.7 pm or more natural fluoride in community water supply, 1969. (U.S. Department of Health, Education and Welfare. Natural Fluoride Content of Community Water Supplies)

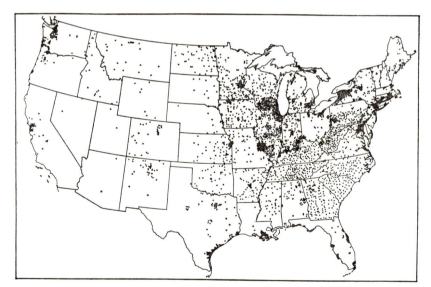

Figure 5. Distribution of communities served with controlled fluoridated water, 1969. Each dot represents a community with controlled fluoridation. (U.S. Department of Health, Education and Welfare. Fluoridation Census 1969)

the tablets are distributed at school approximately 200 times per year, the mean percentage reduction of DMFT scores is 36 percent. As in the case of water fluoridation, the caries inhibition is greater on smooth surfaces than pits and fissures. Interestingly enough, there is also clear evidence for a posteruptive effect, suggesting that fluoride tablets should be kept in the mouth as long as possible.

It is not clear how long protection is maintained after tablet intake is discontinued. Present evidence suggests that a considerable part of the protection is lost when the preventive fluoride supply is suspended.

Finally, it is important to emphasize that dietary fluoride supplements cannot be considered an adequate substitute for community water fluoridation.

Prenatal Fluoride

The question has been raised whether to supplement the diet of pregnant mothers living in a nonfluoride area with fluoride tablets. Experiments using radioactive fluoride have established that the placenta is no true barrier and that the fetus does receive fluoride from the mother's blood. There have been no adequate studies on the cariostatic effectiveness of prenatally administered fluoride tablets; however, some inferential evidence is available by a comparison of the caries in the deciduous teeth of children exposed prenatally and/or postnatally to fluoridated water. Some surveys have claimed an additional protection in the children who received prenatal fluoride in contrast to children with only postnatal fluoride exposure. Others have reported very little effect of prenatal fluoride on the development of caries in deciduous teeth (Table VIII).

Because of the lack of clear-cut response to prenatal fluoride, the Food and Drug Administration considers any fluoride preparation labelled, represented or advertised "for prenatal use" as misbranded and subject to regulatory proceeding. There is no question of safety of these drugs; they are proscribed simply because there is no substantial evi-

TABLE VIII

AVERAGE CARIES PREVALENCE OF 12 DECIDUOUS TEETH
IN 7-YEAR-OLD CHILDREN *

Prenatal Fluoride Exposure	dmft/child	dmfs/child
None	3.43	6.35
<3 mos	3.47	6.70
3–6 mos	3.42	6.20
6–9 mos	3.09	5.72
Full term	3.23	6.02

* Each child had been exposed to postnatal fluoride.

dence of effectiveness in the prevention of dental caries in the offspring.

QUESTIONS FOR DISCUSSION

1. A greater precision in administration of fluoride by tablets has been claimed, compared to water fluoridation because one must drink exactly 1 liter of water fluoridated to 1.0 ppm to obtain the recommended 1 mg of fluoride ion daily. Discuss.

2. Why does fluoride not protect all tooth surfaces equally?

3. If water fluoridation protects teeth by the systemic route, why is there increased caries after defluoridation?

4. Human dietary habits vary considerably in different countries, yet water fluoridation appears to have reduced caries by about the same amount in all the countries where it has been implemented. How can this be?

5. By the beginning of 1972 about 96 million persons in the U.S.A. were receiving optimal amounts of fluoride in their drinking water (either controlled or natural). This represents 59 percent of the population on public water supplies, but only 46 percent of the total population. Using the above information, calculate the number of persons who are not served by public water supplies. What percentage of the total population does this represent? Discuss the significance of this figure.

6. Proponents of milk as a vehicle for fluoride have argued, "Because only milk intended for children will be fluoridated, this method is highly selective. The life-long drink-

ing of fluoride would be avoided." Are these valid reasons for preferring milk rather than water as a means of fluoride ingestion?

7. In a clinical study on the effectiveness of fluoride tablets, three groups of children between 18 and 39 months of age received chewable tablets containing either vitamins, vitamins plus fluoride or fluoride alone. The following data* were obtained:

INCIDENCE OF CARIES IN DECIDUOUS TEETH DURING 2 YEARS

Group	Initial Prevalence Mean defs	Increment Mean defs	Percent Difference
		12 months	
Vitamins	1.35	4.37	....
Vitamins + F	1.81	1.90	−56.5
Fluoride	1.71	1.98	−54.7
		24 months	
Vitamins	0.51	6.93	....
Vitamins + F	1.95	2.39	−65.5
Fluoride	1.03	2.59	−62.6

* Hennon, D.K., Stookey, G.K. and Muhler, J.C.: 1972. Prophylaxis of dental caries: Relative effectiveness of chewable fluoride preparations with and without added vitamins. J. Pediat., *80*:1018–1021.

Discuss these findings.

FURTHER READING

Accepted Dental Therapeutics: 1971. *Council on Dental Therapeutics, American Dental Association,* 34th ed., Chicago, pp. 202–216.

Adler, P.: 1970. Fluorides and dental health. In *Fluorides and Human Health,* W.H.O., Geneva, Switzerland.

Blayney, J.R. and Hill, I.N.: 1967. Fluorine and dental caries. *J. Am. Dent. Assoc., 74*:233–302.

Dunning, J.M.: 1970. *Principles of Dental Public Health,* 2nd ed. Cambridge, Harvard Univ. Press, pp. 231–239, 367–403.

Maier, F.J.: 1963. *Manual of Water Fluoridation Practice.* New York, McGraw Hill.

Maier, F.J.: 1972. *Fluoridation.* Cleveland, CRC Press.

McClure, F.J.: 1962. *Fluoride Drinking Waters.* Public Health Service Publication No. 825.

McClure, F.J.: 1970. *Water fluoridation. The Search and the Victory.* Washington, D.C., U.S. Government Printing Office.

Quimby, F.H. and Bennett, C.C.: 1972. *Fluoridation: A Modern Paradox in Science and Public Policy.* Congressional Res. Serv., Library of Congress.

Young, W.O. and Striffler, D.F.: 1969. *The Dentist, his Practice and his Community,* 2nd ed. Philadelphia, W.B. Saunders, pp. 89–112.

Chapter 2

FLUORIDE DENTIFRICES

S.B. Heifetz and H.S. Horowitz

DENTIFRICE CLASSIFICATION

THE FIRST DENTIFRICE claiming caries-inhibitory properties to receive even so much as provisional acceptance by the Council on Dental Therapeutics of the American Dental Association was one employing stannous fluoride as its active ingredient. This unprecedented action was taken after persuasive and reasonable evidence of the product's effectiveness and safety had been reviewed by the Council. More than ten years have passed since the Council's consequential decision to classify therapeutic dentifrices. During this period, either upon its own initiative or at the request of industry, the Council has undertaken a concerted and continuing effort to thoroughly evaluate various therapeutic dentifrices. Through the experience gained during these years, provisions for the acceptance of therapeutic dentifrices have been established, based upon stringent qualifications and standards with respect to effectiveness, safety, composition and labeling. Starting in 1965, the results of laboratory tests began to receive substantial emphasis in the total evaluatory procedure. However, final acceptance of effectiveness is still dependent on the findings of independent and well-controlled clinical trials in humans.

The Council classifies products in Group A, B, C or D. Group A products are listed in *Accepted Dental Therapeutics* and may use the Seal of Acceptance. Group B products are only provisionally accepted because they lack sufficient evidence to justify an A rating. There is, however, reasonable evidence of usefulness and safety for products in Group B. Group C consists of products for which the evidence is so limited or inconclusive that the products cannot be evaluated accurately. Lastly, Group D products are unacceptable because of their demonstrated inability to meet the standards outlined in the provisions for acceptance.

Decisions of the Council are made after judging all available scientific evidence. Occasionally, some of the supporting materials submitted by manufacturers are in the form of investigators' unpublished manuscripts and restricted documents. Because of the Council's access to special information and its own experience and expertise and that of its consultants in evaluating therapeutic dentifrices, it would be presumptive to attempt to improve upon the reliable information contained in the current edition of *Accepted Dental Therapeutics* and in interim reports that appear periodically in the *Journal of the American Dental Association.* It is recommended, however, that the Council prevail upon investigators and industry to publish promptly the results of a nonconfidential nature that are submitted as supporting evidence.

THERAPEUTIC DENTIFRICES

During the past 30 years, several compounds incorporated in dentifrices have been tested for their caries-inhibitory effect. Field trials with agents such as ammonia and urea compounds and enzyme-inhibitors have yielded, at best, equivocal results. Serious consideration of dentifrices containing penicillin has been mitigated thus far by concern about resistant strains of microorganisms and sensitization of the individual. However, future, successful use of other antibiotics (e.g. tyrothricin, bacitracin) which have little importance in systemic chemotherapy but which are effective in controlling the microorganisms associated with the carious process should not be discounted.

Evaluation of dentifrices containing various compounds of fluoride have been the most widely conducted, and generally these evaluations have yielded encouraging results. The compounds that have attracted the most attention thus far are sodium fluoride, stannous fluoride, sodium monofluoro-phosphate, acid phosphate-fluoride and amine fluoride.

Sodium fluoride was the first agent with fluoride to be incorporated into a conventional toothpaste formulation. Initial clinical studies with dentifrices containing sodium fluoride, however, failed to show a significant reduction in dental caries among participants using the test formulations.

Stannous Fluoride Dentifrices

There followed numerous studies with a dentifrice containing stannous fluoride-calcium pyrophosphate (Crest®). Data on the effectiveness of Crest has generally been consistent, although some of the differences in incremental caries scores between test and control groups have not been statistically significant. Notable differences can be found in the design of these studies, particularly with respect to the frequency of brushing, the extent of brushing instruction and supervision given to the participants and the age of the study subjects. It would be unreasonable, therefore, to expect the findings of these trials to conform closely with each other. Because of the differences in study conditions, it would be inappropriate to compute a combined, overall reduction in dental caries and to use this average as an estimate of the true effectiveness of the stannous fluoride-calcium pyrophosphate dentifrice. The level of conferred protection must be considered in terms of the specific conditions of each study.

Several studies have reported modest reductions in incremental DMF surfaces, on the order of 25 percent or less, following the normal usage at home of a stannous fluoride-calcium pyrophosphate dentifrice. More substantial benefits, a 54 percent reduction in new DMF surfaces, have been observed among groups of students in a military school who were directed to brush three times per day and who received special instruction in oral hygiene. Variation in the frequency of brushing *per se,* however, has not always been found to correlate with the level of protection obtained. In one large-scale dentifrice study it was reported that children who brushed with a stannous fluoride-calcium pyrophosphate toothpaste once a day in school as well as at home derived no additional caries-inhibitory benefits beyond those gained by children who brushed their teeth with the same dentifrice only at home.

Marthaler (1971) has reviewed the data from clinical trials with fluoride compounds published within the past five years. Figures 6 and 7 show the point estimates and attached confidence limits of percentage inhibitions of caries increments obtained from supervised and unsupervised use of fluoride-containing dentifrices. Upon examination of the confidence intervals, he concluded that supervised use generally did not provide appreciably more anticaries protection than under normal home use. In general, small differences between the effectiveness in supervised as compared to unsupervised use were found.

DENTIFRICES, SUPERVISED USE

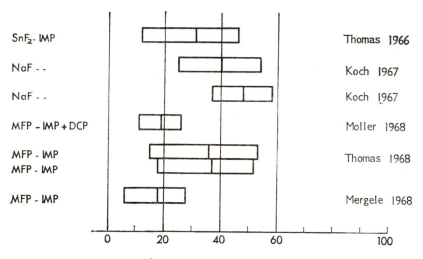

Percent inhibition of increments

Figure 6. Percentage inhibitions of caries increments compared with controls and 95% confidence intervals for each percentage inhibition, compiled from recent clinical trials evaluating the supervised use of fluoride dentifrices.

DENTIFRICES, UNSUPERVISED USE

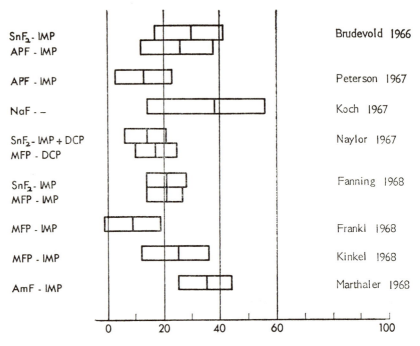

Percent inhibition of increments

Figure 7. Percentage inhibitions of caries increments compared with controls and 95% confidence intervals for each percentage inhibition, compiled from recent clinical trials evaluating the unsupervised use of fluoride dentifrices. SnF₂—stannous fluoride; IMP—insoluble sodium metaphosphate; AFP—acidulated phosphate-fluoride; NaF—sodium fluoride; DCP—dicalcium phosphate; MFP—sodium monofluorophosphate; AmF—amine fluoride. (Courtesy Professor Dr. Marthaler [1971] *Caries Res.*)

Notwithstanding, it is possible that greater effectiveness of a therapeutic dentifrice can be realized when frequent use is accompanied by careful and thorough brushing. This rationale is embodied in the Council on Dental Therapeutics' endorsement of the stannous fluoride-calcium pyrophosphate dentifrice which links protection to a conscientiously applied program of oral hygiene.

Reports of several studies with stannous fluoride dentifrices have shown overall results broken down according to status of tooth eruption. The findings offer evidence that stannous fluoride dentifrices provide more protection to teeth that erupted while a study was in progress than to teeth that were already present when the trial began. Other analyses of data from trials with stannous fluoride dentifrices suggest that greater caries inhibition is produced on proximal (smooth) surfaces than on occlusal or buccolingual (pit and fissure) surfaces.

More tooth pigmentation has been observed in test groups who brushed with stannous fluoride dentifrices than in corresponding controls. However, the frequency and intensity of staining do not appear to be problems of serious concern for the user.

Because of the reactivity of stannous and fluoride ions, it has been difficult to compound compatible dentifrice formulations. Of major concern has been the reaction of ionic fluoride with calcium in the polishing agent to form relatively insoluble calcium fluoride. Research at Indiana University has indicated that calcium pyrophosphate is a compatible polishing agent for use in a stannous fluoride dentifrice. However, results of laboratory studies by others have shown that the availability of ionic fluoride in a stannous fluoride-calcium pyrophosphate dentifrice decreases rapidly when the dentifrice is allowed to age, and when it is stored at elevated temperatures. It has not been established if a corresponding decline in clinical effectiveness of the dentifrice accompanies this partial loss of ionic fluoride. Nevertheless, one may have some reservations about the therapeutic value of tubes of stannous fluoride-calcium pyrophosphate dentifrice that have had an extended shelf-life at greater than room temperatures; a relatively fresh product stored at low temperature theoretically should have the greatest potential for providing maximum protection.

In an attempt to improve upon Crest, several stannous fluoride dentifrices with varying formulations were developed and marketed in the 1960s. Formulations, Cue®, Fact®

and Super Stripe®, all contained insoluble sodium metaphosphate (IMP) as an abrasive, which in laboratory tests showed the property of stabilizing the soluble fractions of tin and fluoride. The three stannous fluoride-IMP dentifrices were classified in Group B by the Council on Dental Therapeutics, whereas the stannous fluoride-calcium pyrophosphate dentifrice has received an A rating. It should be noted that the difference in classification distinguishes between limited (Group B) and extensive (Group A) supporting data and in no way implies superiority. Nevertheless, Cue, Fact and Super Stripe are no longer being manufactured.

Certain aspects of dentifrices with stannous fluoride require further investigation. For example, the duration of benefits has not been established and effectiveness in older persons has not been demonstrated adequately. Observations have been confined mainly to permanent teeth; the effects on deciduous teeth are less definitely known. Corroborative evidence is lacking to indicate that the use of a stannous fluoride dentifrice either in a fluoridated community or in conjunction with other forms of stannous fluoride therapy will provide additive benefits.

Sodium Fluoride Dentifrices

It has been hypothesized that stannous fluoride dentifrices have been successful and the initially developed sodium fluoride dentifrices were not because the former have more compatible abrasive formulations and lower pH values; low acidity tends to favor the deposition of fluoride in enamel. Support for this hypothesis is offered by findings of recent clinical studies with a sodium fluoride dentifrice formulated with orthophosphoric acid and a calcium-free abrasive, insoluble sodium metaphosphate. Children brushing with the new formulation had significantly less new decay than subjects in the control groups. However, it appears that a sodium fluoride dentifrice containing a compatible abrasive but lacking a low pH can also be effective in reducing incremental decay, as shown by findings of clinical tests in Sweden and Canada. The product evaluated in the Canadian dentifrice trial had a neutral pH and contained calcium pyrophosphate as the abrasive (Gleem® - NaF or Gleem II®, see Table IX). Although these reports of newer sodium fluoride dentifrices are encouraging, meaningful evaluation of these products must await the completion of more studies.

Monofluorophosphate Dentifrice

In the past few years, reports have been published on a dentifrice with sodium monofluorophosphate which uses insoluble sodium metaphosphate as an abrasive (Colgate with MFP®, see Table IX). Clinical trials with the dentifrice have been conducted by several investigators, under conditions of supervised and unsupervised use, with varying frequencies of brushing. In all the trials, some degree of effectiveness has been reported, and generally the benefits have been statistically significant. It has been reported that the monofluorophosphate dentifrice gave greater protection than the stannous fluoride-calcium pyrophosphate

TABLE IX
COMPOSITION OF FLUORIDE DENTIFRICES

Component	Procter & Gamble[1] Crest		Colgate Palmolive[2] Colgate MFP		Procter & Gamble[3] Gleem II	
Therapeutic compound	SnF_2	0.4%	Na_2FPO_3	0.76%	NaF	0.22%
Abrasive	$Ca_2P_2O_7$	39%	$(NaPO_3)_x$	41.8%	$Ca_2P_2O_7$	40.0%
	$Sn_2P_2O_7$	1%	$CaHPO_4$	5.0%		
Humectant	Glycerol	10%	Glycerol	12.8%	Glycerol	30.0%
	Sorbitol	20%	Sorbitol	14.0%	Sorbitol	
Binder					Sod. carboxy methyl Cellulose & Veegum	1.5%
Water		25%		19.4%		26.1%
Detergent			Lauryl Sarcosinate	2.0%	Sod. monoglyc sulf. & sod. alkylsulfonate	1.0%
Miscellaneous		4.6%		4.2%		1.18%

[1] *J.A.D.A. 69*:195, 1964—Council on Dental Therapeutics Group A
[2] *J.A.D.A. 79*:937, 1969—Council on Dental Therapeutics Group A
[3] Schrotenboer, G.H., Secretary—Council on Dental Therapeutics, Personal Communication

dentifrice when tested in the same studies. However, these studies lacked a true control group, and therefore it was not possible to determine the absolute level of protection conferred by either product. It has also been reported that the teeth of children in groups who brushed with the mono-fluorophosphate dentifrice have exhibited less staining than those of children who used a stannous fluoride dentifrice. On the basis of positive clinical evidence from eight studies, the Council on Dental Therapeutics classified Colgate with MFP as a product in Group A. The lack of staining associated with the use of a dentifrice with monofluorophosphate may give the product some advantage over stannous fluoride dentifrices in gaining acceptability.

Aminohydrofluoride Dentifrices

In vitro experiments indicate that organic amine hydrofluoride may provide better protection than simple inorganic salts of fluoride in protecting enamel from decalcification by acid and in preventing bacterial plaque formation. Results of studies in animals show that it is possible to incorporate amine fluorides into dentifrices without loss of cariostatic activity. Clinical findings of a study extending over seven years suggest that long-term inhibition of dental decay (about 30%) can be obtained from unsupervised use of the dentifrice. The dentifrice contained two amine fluoride compounds, diethanol aminopropyl-N-ethanol octadecylamine-dihydrofluoride and cetylamine hydrofluoride.

$$\left[CH_3(CH_2)_{17}\!-\!\underset{\underset{\displaystyle CH_2CH_2OH}{|}}{N}\!-\!(CH_2)_3\!-\!N\!\!\begin{array}{c} CH_2CH_2OH \\ CH_2CH_2OH \end{array} \right] \cdot 2HF$$

Diethanol aminopropyl-N-ethanol octadecylamine-dihydrofluoride

$$CH_3(CH_2)_{15}NH_3{}^+F^-$$
cetylamine hydrofluoride

Both substances have in common a long aliphatic chain, with 16 or 18 carbon atoms, which is responsible for the dentifrice's property of lowering surface tension. Further investigation of the organic amine hydrofluorides is indicated.

SUMMARY

There is little doubt that new and better dentifrices will continue to be developed. Existing therapeutic dentifrices, however, that have been classified as effective by the Council on Dental Therapeutics of the American Dental Association provide limited protection against the development of dental caries, and therefore the public should be encouraged to use these products. However, because therapeutic dentifrices are commercially produced, information about their caries-preventive properties is more than adequately disseminated by the manufacturers. The intense commercial advertising of therapeutic dentifrices obviates the need for additional, active promotion by public health agencies.

QUESTIONS FOR DISCUSSION

1. What are some of the factors that may account for the variations in the magnitude of effectiveness reported in studies of stannous fluoride dentifrices?

2. There are persons in the dental field who deplore the decision of the Council on Dental Therapeutics to classify therapeutic dentifrices. What is your position on the wisdom of this action and why?

3. The Finn and Jamison Study is an example of a clinical trial in which the experimental dentifrices are compared with an *active control* (a dentifrice conceded to have therapeutic value), rather than with a conventional, inactive control. Discuss the merits and weaknesses of this type of study design.

4. The following dentifrice formulation has been patented:

Ingredient	% Composition
Silica Cleansing & Polishing Agent	12.00
Insoluble Sodium Metaphosphate	6.00
Silica Thickening Agent	5.00
Sodium Carragheenate	1.30
Saccharin	0.20
Glycerin	31.53
Water	32.95
Polyethylene Glycol	4.00
Colorant (1% solution)	0.02
Flavor	0.90
Hexachlorophene	0.05
Tribromosalicylanilide	0.05
Sodium-Lauryl Sulfate-Glycerine Mixture (21%)	6.00

Discuss the purpose of the various ingredients. Do you think this dentifrice merits a clinical trial for caries prevention?

FURTHER READING

Bixler, D. and Muhler, J.C.: 1966. Effectiveness of a stannous fluoride-containing dentifrice in reducing dental caries in children in a boarding school environment. *J. Am. Dent. Assoc., 72*:653–658.

Brudevold, F. and Chilton, N.W.: 1966. Comparative study of a fluoride dentifrice containing soluble phosphate and a calcium-free abrasive. Second-year report. *J. Am. Dent. Assoc., 72*:889–894.

Duckworth, R.: 1968. Fluoride dentifrices. A review of clinical trials in the United Kingdom. *Br. Dent. J., 124*:505–509.

Fanning, E.A., Gotjamanos, T. and Vourles, N.J.: 1968. The use of fluoride dentifrices in the control of dental caries: Methodology and results of clinical trial. *Aust. Dent. J., 13*:201–206.

Finn, S.B. and Jamison, H.C.: 1963. A comparative clinical study of three dentifrices. *J. Dent. Child., 30*:17–25.

Frankl, S.N. and Alman, J.E.: 1968. Report of a 3-year clinical trial comparing a toothpaste containing sodium monofluorophosphate with 2 marketed products. *J. Oral Ther., 4*:443–450.

Grön, P. and Brudevold, F.: 1967. The effectiveness of NaF dentifrices. *J. Dent. Child., 34*:122–127.

Horowitz, H.S., Law, F.E., Thompson, M. B. and Chamberlin, S.R.: 1966. Evaluation of a stannous fluoride dentifrice for use in dental public health programs. I. Basic findings. *J. Am. Dent. Assoc., 72*:408–422.

Kinkel, H. and Stolte, G.: 1968. Zur Wirking einer natrium fluorophosphat— und brom chlorophenhaltigen Zahnpasta in chronischen Tierexperiment und auf die Karies bei Kinderwährend eines 2 Jahre langen unüberwachten Gebrauches. *Dtsch. Zahnarztebe, 9*:455–460.

Koch, G.: 1967. Effect of sodium fluoride in dentifrice and mouthwash on incidence of dental caries in school children. *Odontol. Revy.,* vol. 18, suppl. 12.

Marthaler, T.M.: 1968. Caries-inhibition after seven years of unsupervised use of an amine fluoride dentifrice. *Br. Dent. J., 124*:510–515.

Marthaler, T.M.: 1971. Confidence limits of results of clinical tests with fluoride administration. *Caries Res., 4*:343–372.

Mergele, M.E.: 1968. Report I. A supervised brushing study in State institutional schools. *Bull. Acad. Med. New Jersey, 14*:247–250.

Möller, I.J., Holst, J.J. and Sorensen, E.: 1968. Caries reducing effect of a sodium monofluorophosphate dentifrice. *Br. Dent. J., 124*:209–213.

Naylor, M.N. and Emslie, R.D.: 1967. Clinical testing of stannous fluoride and sodium monofluorophosphate dentifrices in London school children. *Br. Dent. J., 123*:17–23.

Peterson, J.K. and Williamson, L.: 1967. Field test of a sodium fluoride dentifrice containing acid orthophosphate and insoluble metaphosphate abrasive. *J. Oral Ther., 4*:1–4.

Thomas, A.E. and Jamison, H.C.: 1966. Effect of SnF_2 dentifrices on caries in children. 2-year clinical study of supervised brushing in children's homes. *J. Am. Dent. Assoc., 23*:844–852.

Thomas, A.E. and Jamison, H.C.: 1968. Effect of a combination of 2 cariostatic agents in children: 2-year clinical study of supervised brushing in children's homes. *J. Am. Dent. Assoc., 81*:118–125.

Chapter 3

THE CURRENT STATUS OF TOPICAL FLUORIDES IN PREVENTIVE DENTISTRY

HERSCHEL S. HOROWITZ AND STANLEY B. HEIFETZ

HUNDREDS OF clinical studies conducted during the past 25 years have evaluated the use of topical fluorides in protecting the enamel surface of teeth from caries attack. These investigations have led to the development of the various topical fluoride procedures that are available today. This chapter summarizes current knowledge on the subject by reviewing pertinent studies and by pinpointing the conclusions they support. This material should be helpful to dental personnel and dental health agencies in their promotional efforts in preventive dentistry and in developing and managing the increasing number of comprehensive dental programs for children.

TOPICAL FLUORIDE SOLUTIONS

Sodium Fluoride

The recommended treatment technic for the application of a solution of sodium fluoride begins with cleaning the clinical crowns of the teeth, with use of a standard prophylaxis paste in a motor-driven rubber cup. After the prophylaxis, an upper and opposing lower quadrant (half the mouth at a time) are isolated with cotton rolls held in appropriate holders and the teeth are dried thoroughly with a stream of compressed air. A 2% sodium fluoride solution is applied to the teeth with cotton applicators so that all surfaces are made visibly wet. The solution is permitted to dry for about three minutes. Second, third, and fourth applications, not preceded by prophylaxes, are given at intervals of approximately one week. As with all topically applied fluoride agents, caries inhibition presumably begins as soon as treatment is completed. The series of treatments is recommended at ages three, seven, 11, and 13. These ages were selected so that fluoride is applied shortly after the eruption of groups of teeth, thus minimizing the time that teeth are at risk from caries attack before treatment. The ages should be varied, if possible, with each child's individual pattern of tooth eruption.

The procedure for the application of sodium fluoride was developed by Knutson and co-workers, who tested different fluoride solutions, concentrations and frequencies of application in a series of large-scale studies involving thousands of school children. In summary, results of these early studies indicated that (1) a minimum of four applications with a 2 percent sodium fluoride solution appears to give the maximum effect—a reduction of about 40 percent in new carious teeth; (2) increasing the interval between individual applications in the series from about one week to three to six months decreases the effectiveness of treatment; and (3) omission of a prophylaxis preceding the series of treatments reduces the benefits by about half.

Studies conducted throughout the world by other investigators have confirmed the caries-preventive properties of topically applied sodium fluoride. A variety of technics of application have been tested, but the procedure developed by the U.S. Public Health Service has been the most widely used, and it appears to be the most reliable. A review of the literature reveals an impressive number of studies that have essentially duplicated the results obtained by Knutson and his co-workers. In spite of some variation, 30 to 40 percent reductions in dental caries incidence in the permanent teeth of children living in an area with insufficient levels of fluoride in the water supply have been reported quite consistently.

Certain aspects of the potential usefulness of topically

applied sodium fluoride need further investigation. More long-term studies must be done to determine precisely how long after treatment sodium fluoride continues to exert a beneficial effect; results of some investigations suggest that a falloff in effectiveness may occur in less than three years, yet there is little evidence to indicate that greater benefits can be derived when the series of four applications is repeated annually rather than at the specified ages.

Reports of a few studies that have tested a 2% sodium fluoride solution applied to deciduous teeth have shown reductions in the incidence of dental caries ranging from 22 to 40 percent. On the other hand, studies that evaluated the effectiveness of sodium fluoride applications in adult populations offer conflicting data. Two investigations in adults reported reductions of about 50 percent, whereas two other studies obtained negative results.

Particular advantages and disadvantages are associated with the use of a 2% sodium fluoride solution. It is relatively stable when kept in a plastic container and there is no need to prepare a fresh solution for each patient. The taste is well accepted by patients. The solution is nonirritating to the gingiva and does not cause discoloration of tooth structure or silicate fillings. Once applied to the teeth, the solution is allowed to dry for three minutes; thus the clinician in public health programs can pursue a multiple-chair procedure. The series of treatments must be repeated only four times in the general age range of three to 17, rather than at annual or semiannual intervals; therefore, in a public health program, other groups of children can be treated in intervening years. The major disadvantage of the use of sodium fluoride is that the patient must make four visits to the dentist within a relatively short time.

Stannous Fluoride

The recommended procedure for the topical application of stannous fluoride begins with a thorough prophylaxis.

Each tooth surface is carefully cleaned and polished with pumice for five to ten seconds. The pumice is carried between the teeth with unwaxed dental floss and the proximal surfaces of the teeth are stripped. The teeth are then isolated with cotton rolls and dried with compressed air. Either a quadrant or half of the mouth can be treated at one time, depending on the operator's ability to keep the teeth completely free of saliva. A freshly prepared 8% solution of stannous fluoride is applied continually to the teeth with cotton applicators, so that the teeth are kept moist with the solution for four minutes. This usually means a reapplication to a particular tooth every 15 to 30 seconds.

The recommended frequency of stannous fluoride treatments after the initial application depends on the patient's susceptibility to dental caries. In highly susceptible patients, the dentist should repeat the application at least once every six months. If the patient is not particularly caries prone, a single treatment can be given once a year.

No additional anticariogenic benefit is derived from a second application of an 8% stannous fluoride solution given within a day or two after the first application provided. Four semiannual applications of a 10% solution of stannous fluoride applied for 30 seconds has produced benefits, after two years, equal to those produced by the traditional four-minute application of an 8% solution.

Much of the work dealing with the effectiveness of stannous fluoride has been conducted by Muhler and his associates at the University of Indiana. This group of investigators has reported many times that annual or semiannual applications of an 8% stannous fluoride solution produce a statistically significant decrease in the development of new dental caries. A composite of the results of their studies indicates benefits with the use of stannous fluoride exceeding the 30 to 40 percent figures generally accepted for a 2% sodium fluoride solution. Levels of protection ranging from 47 to 78 percent fewer new DMF surfaces among treated children have been reported in these studies.

Other investigators also have found stannous fluoride to be effective. However, the magnitude of the benefits reported by others has generally been less than that obtained by Muhler and his co-workers. Peterson and Williamson (1962) reported a 26 percent lower increment in DMF teeth after two yearly applications of an 8% stannous fluoride solution. Law, Jeffries, and Sheary (1961) found, with use of the half-mouth technic, that a single application of an 8% solution of stannous fluoride produced a reduction of approximately 17 percent in the development of new carious teeth after one year. Harris (1963) reported that semiannual half-mouth applications of an 8% solution of stannous fluoride to children resulted in a 23 percent reduction in new lesions.

Several other studies have been conducted on the effectiveness of a topically applied stannous fluoride solution under various conditions. Findings on adults and on deciduous teeth showed the agent to be effective. Decay-preventive benefits ranging from 27 to 75% reductions in DMF surfaces were also demonstrated after the use of a stannous fluoride solution in combination with other preventive agents containing the stannous and fluoride ions.

On the other hand, in conflict with the many favorable reports, a few recent studies evaluating stannous fluoride have shown the agent to possess little or no anticariogenic properties. In a study by Wellock and others (1965), the application of an 8% stannous fluoride solution to the teeth of children failed to reduce incremental dental caries after one year.

Negative results with stannous fluoride were obtained in Sweden by Torell and Ericsson (1965) in a two-year study designed to evaluate the caries-reducing effects of various methods of fluoride application. No reduction was observed in a group of children who received two annual topical applications of a 10% stannous fluoride solution.

The results of a study conducted by Horowitz and Lucye (1966) showed that children who were treated annually for two years with an 8% stannous fluoride solution failed to demonstrate any decay preventive effect after either the first or the second year.

One major advantage in using an 8% stannous fluoride solution at six- to 12-month intervals is that this frequency conforms to practicing dentists' usual patient-recall system. If the preventive procedure can be completed in one appointment, the necessity of frequent visits is eliminated. Administrative difficulties, particularly in public health programs, created by the need to arrange four appointments (as for sodium fluoride applications) are avoided. The recommended scheduling for stannous fluoride topical applications has the advantage of permitting teeth to be treated soon after eruption when they are highly susceptible to fluoride incorporation and before they have had a chance to decay.

Stannous fluoride also has several disadvantages. In aqueous solution the material is not stable; it undergoes fairly rapid hydrolysis and oxidation and forms stannous hydroxide and the stannic ion. This reaction reduces the agent's effectiveness. Consequently, a fresh solution must be prepared for each treatment. Because an 8% solution is quite astringent and disagreeable in taste, its application is unpleasant. Unfortunately, the addition of flavoring agents to mask the unpleasant taste of stannous fluoride is contraindicated. The solution occasionally causes a reversible tissue irritation, manifested by gingival blanching. The reaction usually occurs in individuals with poor gingival health.

Pigmentation of teeth after the topical application of stannous fluoride solutions has been reported by many investigators. The pigmentation has a characteristic light brown color; it usually appears in association with carious lesions and hypocalcified regions of the teeth and around the margins of restorations. Some investigators believe that the stannous ion in stannous fluoride plays an important role in determining the anticariogenic potential of the agent. Muhler (1966) maintains that once a pre-carious or carious area becomes pigmented (with the stannous ion), the lesion will fail to increase in size. Some data, however, suggest that the presence of tin in teeth has little protective effect. Differences of opinion also exist on the extent and significance of the staining produced by stannous fluoride.

Because topically applied stannous fluoride produces pigmentation of teeth, it is difficult to measure dental caries in test and control groups at the same level of detection. Similarly, a masking of lesions on radiographs by the tin moiety of stannous fluoride has been reported. Both these phenomena would tend to cause the assessment of dental caries in a clinical trial to be biased and may partly explain the wide divergence in findings that has been reported with topically applied stannous fluoride.

There appears to be adequate evidence to show that four-minute applications of 8% solutions of stannous fluoride can produce protection against dental caries. It would be desirable, however, if additional investigations were conducted in which special precautions were taken to give participants a thorough prophylaxis before each follow-up examination in order to minimize possible bias. If these studies were positive and further research showed that there was no masking of carious lesions on radiographs of persons treated with stannous fluoride, doubts concerning the efficacy of stannous fluoride would be dispelled.

Acidulated Phosphate-fluoride

The preferred procedure for applying acidulated phosphate-fluoride solution, a relatively new agent containing 1.23% fluoride, is the same as that for stannous fluoride except that an acidulated phosphate-fluoride solution is stable when kept in plastic containers, and thus a fresh solution need not be prepared for each patient.

Initial clinical studies which evaluated topical applications of acidulated phosphate-fluoride indicated that it might possess anticariogenic properties surpassing those of agents already in use. At the end of one 2-year study with annual applications, children in a test group demonstrated a 67 percent smaller increment in DMF teeth and a 70 percent reduction in DMF surfaces compared with the untreated controls. In another investigation, a traditional 2% sodium fluoride solution was applied to half the mouth and a 2% sodium fluoride solution acidulated with orthophosphoric acid was applied to the other half. Results indicated that the half treated with the acid phosphate solution had about 50 percent fewer new carious lesions than the half treated with neutral sodium fluoride. The difference in increment was reported to be highly significant.

The beneficial effects found in more recent studies evaluating the topical application of acidulated phosphate-fluoride solutions have tended to be smaller than those obtained in the initial studies, but the newer findings nevertheless have been encouraging. Wellock and others (1965) reported that, at the end of two years, children treated annually with the acidulated phosphate-fluoride solution had 44 percent fewer new DMF teeth and 52 percent fewer new DMF surfaces compared with children in a control group. Cartwright and his co-workers (1968) obtained a 49 percent reduction in DMF tooth increments in children who had received four semiannual applications of the solution.

Horowitz (1968, 1969) has reported annual results of a three-year study designed to test the caries-inhibiting effect of an acidulated phosphate-fluoride solution and gel. After three years, children who received traditionally applied annual applications of a flavored acidulated phosphate-fluoride solution experienced 28 percent fewer new DMF surfaces than the controls. Children who had been given semiannual applications of the solution developed 41 percent fewer DMF surfaces than the controls after three years. Application of the agent in gel form via a wax tray produced a 24 percent reduction in DMF surfaces of test groups as compared with the controls. Mean incremental DMF surface scores for children in each of the three test groups were significantly different from those in the control group. It was concluded from these findings that both acidulated phosphate-fluoride solution and gel are effective cariostatic agents.

Another evaluation of the cariostatic effectiveness of an acidulated phosphate-fluoride solution and gel was done on children treated with the gel in wax or foam rubber trays. At the end of two years a 41 percent reduction in incremental DMF surfaces compared with children in the control group was demonstrated. However, application of the solution in the traditional manner or by means of a tray technic resulted in minimal, nonsignificant reductions in new DMF surfaces of 11 and 13 percent respectively.

A study of professionally applied acidulated phosphate-fluoride gel reported no difference, after one year, in the incidence of carious lesions between a group who received an application of the gel in wax trays and a control group that was given a placebo. Another study found, after one year, 28 percent fewer new DMF surfaces among children eight to 12 years old who had received a single application of acidulated phosphate-fluoride gel applied in foam rubber trays, compared with controls.

Acidulated phosphate-fluoride is reported to have none of the disadvantages of sodium or stannous fluoride. The solution is stable if kept in plastic containers, causes no discoloration of the teeth, is nonirritating to the gingiva, and has an acceptable taste. Single annual applications are recommended.

Results obtained to date with a 1.23% acidulated phosphate-fluoride solution, although subject to some variations, nevertheless provide ample evidence to document the therapeutic value of the agent in reducing the incidence of dental caries. However, further investigations are needed to determine the exact degree of caries protection conferred by the solution and the best method and frequency of applying it. Additional investigations should be made with the acidulated phosphate-fluoride gel to compare its efficacy with that of the solution.

Stannous Hexafluorozirconate

Researchers at Indiana University have developed a new compound, stannous hexafluorozirconate ($SnZrF_6$) which according to *in vitro* and *in vivo* studies is said to be effective in reducing the solubility of enamel and in preventing dental caries. Results of two preliminary investigations with children who received semiannual topical applications of stannous hexafluorozirconate showed decided reductions in the incidence of dental caries. In one trial, one-minute topical applications of 16% stannous hexafluorozirconate at six-month intervals produced caries reductions in DMF surfaces of 96 percent after nine months. In the other study, a 76 percent lower incidence of new DMF surfaces was achieved with semiannual treatments of 24% $SnZrF_6$ after 12 months. However, the number and magnitude of negative incremental caries scores that appear in the tabular data are disconcerting.

Toxic reactions after the use of stannous hexafluorozirconate in a zirconium silicate prophylaxis paste have been reported. The Food and Drug Administration has requested of the sponsor that no further studies be initiated until adequate preclinical studies have been performed to demonstrate safety.

FLUORIDE PROPHYLAXIS PASTES

The successful addition of fluoride to commercial toothpaste suggested that fluoride could also be incorporated into a prophylaxis paste as another means of caries control. Inasmuch as a dental prophylaxis is prescribed to precede a topical application of fluoride, a saving in treatment time and effort would result if the two procedures could be accomplished simultaneously by the use of a therapeutic, fluoride-containing prophylaxis paste alone. It is also possible that a prophylaxis paste and topical solution, each containing fluoride, would produce an additive effect, thus justifying their combined use.

The use of a fluoride prophylaxis paste can be traced back to 1946, when a paste containing 1% sodium fluoride was evaluated in a small group of children. Caries reductions of from 25 to 43 percent were reported, depending on the number of treatments. However, these results in a replicate study with use of a larger sample were not confirmed.

The United States Air Force and Indiana University have each developed a stannous fluoride prophylaxis paste. The Air Force formulation, a stable silicone paste, uses silex as the abrasive. Peterson, Jordan, and Snyder (1963) carried out a two-year clinical evaluation of the stannous fluoride-silex-silicone prophylaxis paste used once a year and twice a year and also used once a year with a follow-up topical application of an 8% stannous fluoride solution. They reported a 34 percent decrease in new DMF surfaces for the group receiving annual treatments with the paste and a 42 percent reduction after seminannual applications. However, the group that received the annual stannous fluoride prophylaxis followed by a stannous fluoride solution did not experience lower increments of decay than the group treated with only the stannous fluoride paste. Hennon and Muhler (1962) found the silex-silicone-fluoride paste to be seriously lacking as a material for cleaning and polishing teeth satisfactorily.

An aqueous stannous fluoride-lava pumice prophylaxis paste developed at Indiana University has been used on American Indian children living in North Dakota. The paste tasted better, cleaned better, and was less irritating to the gingiva than the silex-silicone-stannous fluoride paste.

Bixler and Muhler (1964) reported average reductions of 34 percent in DMF tooth and surface increments at the end of one year in a group of children who had received semiannual treatments of the stannous fluoride-lava pumice prophylaxis paste. Another group in the same study was treated with the paste followed by an 8% stannous fluoride topical application; this group demonstrated even greater benefits. Results after two years and three years showed that the agents continued to maintain their effectiveness.

Reductions ranging from 27 to 61 percent in DMF surface increments have been reported with U.S. Navy enlisted men after two years in groups receiving a stannous fluoride-lava pumice prophylaxis paste in conjunction with a 0.4% stannous fluoride dentifrice, a 10% stannous fluoride solution, or both. However, in a group treated with only the stannous fluoride-lava pumice prophylaxis paste, a minimal reduction (12% fewer DMF surfaces) was reported.

Horowitz and Lucye (1966) failed to replicate the findings of the Indiana group of investigators with respect to the efficacy of the stannous fluoride-lava pumice prophylaxis paste. After two years, children who received annual prophylaxes with the stannous fluoride paste showed similar incremental caries scores to those of children in the control group. The investigators also observed no caries protection after combined treatment with the stannous fluoride paste and an 8% stannous fluoride solution.

Because of the equivocal findings of the few studies evaluating the benefits of a stannous fluoride-lava pumice prophylaxis paste, judgment of this agent's therapeutic efficacy must be reserved until positive results of additional investigations are reported.

Recently, two new therapeutic prophylaxis pastes became available commercially—an acidulated phosphate fluoride-silicon dioxide prophylaxis paste and a stannous fluoride-zirconium silicate prophylaxis paste. No reports of studies evaluating the professional application of the stannous fluoride-zirconium silicate prophylaxis paste could be located in the literature. *In vitro* laboratory data show that exposure to acidulated phosphate fluoride-silicon dioxide paste produces an uptake of fluoride by enamel as great as that from exposure to an acidulated phosphate-fluoride solution. However, findings to document the clinical efficacy of the new paste are lacking.

A two-year study on children in both a fluoridated and a nonfluoridated community has been conducted to determine the caries inhibitory effectiveness of freshly prepared acidulated phosphate fluoride-lava pumice prophylactic paste. The paste was applied annually. Two examiners independently examined the entire study population; both consistently found only slightly smaller caries increments in the treated groups than in the control groups in both communities. The authors suggested that the minimal caries inhibition observed might be attributed to the neutralization of the acid phosphate-fluoride solution in the paste by the pumice abrasive.

SELF-ADMINISTRATION OF TOPICAL FLUORIDES

The traditional approach to the administration of topical fluorides for the prevention of dental decay requires that each child be treated individually by a dentist or dental hygienist and that special equipment and facilities be used. Although professionally applied topical fluorides are well adapted for use in private dental practice, the method has disadvantages for public health programs in which preventive benefits are sought for many children. The increasing shortage of professional dental manpower and the relatively high cost of treatments accentuate the shortcomings of a professionally administered technic as a public health measure.

In the search for methods to overcome these drawbacks, several investigators have evaluated various self-administration procedures for the application of topical fluorides.

In Sweden, elementary school children brushed their teeth with a 1% sodium fluoride solution. During a two-year period, the children made nine applications in school under the supervision of a school dental health officer. Data showed that children in the test group developed 16 percent fewer carious teeth in their maxillary arches than did children in the control group. No clear-cut benefits for teeth in the lower jaw were found.

Another study was conducted to test the caries-inhibiting effect of self-administered solutions of sodium fluoride, zirconium fluoride, and ferric fluoride. An evaluation was made of each solution applied at frequencies of two and five brushings per year. At the end of two years, a comparison of results between the control and test groups indicated that five annual applications of the sodium fluoride and ferric fluoride solutions provided significant reductions of 29 and 33 percent respectively in the proportion of previously sound permanent teeth that became carious, whereas five applications of zirconium fluoride produced a 17 percent reduction. Two annual applications of any of the agents produced either minimal or no reductions compared with the control group.

In a fluoridated community, Goaz and others (1963, 1966) investigated the anticariogenic effectiveness of daily brushing at home with a 6% sodium monofluorophosphate solution. After nine and 14 months, children in the test group showed a significantly lower relative increment of decay (RID) and number of new decayed and filled surfaces (ΔDFS) than children in the control group. After 21 months, both methods of assessment showed approximately a 50 percent reduction in the rate of decay. Unfortunately, the use of relatively uncommon caries indexes and an inordinately high number of reported reversals in diagnosis make the results difficult to interpret. No adequate clinical studies of topical application of fluorophosphate solution have been reported. This is surprising inasmuch as many studies with sodium monofluorophosphate have been done in laboratory animals, and the agent has been successfully incorporated in a commercial dentifrice.

A study was conducted in Canada to determine whether an acidulated phosphate-fluoride solution used four or five times per year in a classroom toothbrushing drill would measurably reduce the incidence of dental caries. After one year, children in the test group had 38 percent fewer new DMF surfaces than the controls. Second-year results were less favorable; the experimental group had 15 percent fewer new lesions than the control group.

The U.S. Navy is currently conducting a large-scale program that uses a partly self-administered technic for topical fluoride application. The treatment consists of a supervised toothbrushing by the participants with an 8.9% stannous fluoride-lava pumice prophylaxis paste, the application of a 10% stannous fluoride solution for a minimum of 15 seconds by a trained operator, and the use at home of a stannous fluoride calcium pyrophosphate dentifrice. After one year, the Navy enlisted men who followed the three-step procedure showed reductions in incremental dental caries of approximately 50 percent compared with subjects in the control group. It is difficult to reconcile these results with those obtained by Horowitz and Lucye (1966), in which the same stannous fluoride-lava pumice prophylaxis paste and an 8% stannous fluoride solution professionally applied to the teeth of children yielded no protection against incremental caries.

Muhler (1968) has reviewed the results of several unpublished pilot studies with a self-administered stannous fluoride-zirconium silicate prophylactic paste. However, it is not possible to comment validly on the reported effectiveness of the new agent-technic because only brief descriptions of the studies and incomplete summary data are presented in the review paper.

In 1970, Muhler and others published the first full report of a clinical study evaluating the effectiveness of the stannous fluoride-zirconium silicate prophylactic paste. Children in the Virgin Islands gave themselves a single self-application of the agent under the supervision of a dentist or dental hygienist. After one year, those children who brushed with the zirconium silicate paste containing 9% stannous fluoride had developed an average of 1.24 fewer DMF surfaces than children who used a placebo paste. The reduction of 64 percent in new DMF surfaces was statistically significant despite a large loss of subjects, particularly in the test group.

Based on the initial promising work with the stannous fluoride-zirconium silicate paste done under the auspices of Indiana University, Gunz (1971) carried out a study to confirm the paste's decay-preventive properties. Children in the test group self-applied the stannous fluoride-zirconium silicate paste according to the recommended technic. A supply of zirconium silicate paste without stannous fluoride was provided by Indiana University for use by children in the control group. Fourteen months following a single self-application, incremental DF scores of children in the test and control groups were the same for all practical clinical purposes, 2.38 and 2.58 surfaces respectively. In previous studies by Indiana University reporting benefits after a single self-application of the paste, follow-up examinations had been made 12 months after application. It is extremely doubtful, however, that the slightly greater length of Gunz' study could explain the lack of confirmatory findings.

Heifetz and others (1970) undertook a study to determine the efficacy of a self-administered tooth brushing procedure with acidulated phosphate-fluoride. Under the supervision of lay personnel, children in the study brushed their teeth in school with the agent approximately once every two months. Findings after two years were disappointing; the data failed to show a decay-preventive effect from brushing with a 0.6% acidulated phosphate-fluoride solution either with or without a prior prophylaxis or with a 1.23% acidulated phosphate-fluoride gel. It appears that a frequency of application greater than once every two months may be necessary to obtain appreciable benefits from self-administration of the materials tested.

In a pilot study in 1946 on fluoride mouthwash, a small group of dental students was instructed to use either a sodium acetate-acetic acid mouthwash containing 0.01% sodium fluoride with a pH of 4 or a nonfluoride mouthwash at least three times a week. The findings after one year failed to indicate that the users of the acidulated fluoride mouthwash derived any appreciable dental benefits. Because the findings were based on observations of only a few participants, the authors said that no definite conclusions about the effectiveness of the fluoride mouthwash could be drawn.

No reduction in new decayed or filled (DF) teeth or surfaces was found using a 0.01% acidulated sodium fluoride mouthwash (pH 4) twice weekly by youngsters for one year.

Compared with these negative findings are the promising results of more recent work conducted in Sweden with caries-prophylactic mouthwashes. Children who had rinsed their mouths under supervision once every other week with either a 0.2% neutral sodium fluoride solution or an iron fluoride solution showed "significant reductions" in dental caries after one year.

On the basis of this report, a study to evaluate further the effectiveness of a fluoride mouthwash in reducing dental caries was conducted. Children rinsed their teeth once a month in school with a neutral 0.2% sodium fluoride solution under the supervision of a dental nurse. The effectiveness of the procedure was assessed by comparing the percentages of children who received new fillings after using the fluoride mouthrinse for one year with corresponding data on record for untreated children. Significantly lower percentages of children, ranging from 13 to 27 percent, received (and ostensibly required) care after use of the mouthwash.

Because both the Swedish studies employed unorthodox methods to evaluate the effects of treatment statistically, it is difficult to interpret fully the reported benefits. The measurement of overall differences in incremental caries based solely on data from dental care received lacks desirable precision.

Torell and Ericsson (1965) have reported results of a clinical trial testing various methods of topical fluoride application. Included among the evaluated procedures were a daily unsupervised rinsing at home (after the evening toothbrushing) with a neutral 0.05% sodium fluoride solution and, under the supervision of dental nurses, a fortnightly mouth-rinsing at school with a neutral 0.2% sodium fluoride solution. At the conclusion of the two-year study, children in the daily mouth-rinsing group showed a 50 percent reduction in mean incremental caries scores compared with children in the control group. Lesser benefits—a 21 percent reduction in average new DMF surfaces—were found in children who rinsed fortnightly. The difference in caries protection afforded by the two mouth-rinsing procedures was statistically significant; this indicates the importance of frequent application in enhancing the effect of topically applied fluorides. Compared with the findings for other groups in the study who received professionally administered fluoride applications or who brushed with fluoride dentifrices, the daily mouth-washing procedure also yielded significantly better results.

In a feasibility study on the use of a stannous fluoride mouthwash in a school preventive dentistry program, the control group rinsed daily with a placebo mouthwash and the test group followed the same procedure, using a 0.1% stannous fluoride mouthwash. Clinical evaluations made after a treatment period of only five months showed that children in the test group developed 30.5 percent fewer carious surfaces than children in the control group. The reduction, however, was not statistically significant, a finding that was not unexpected, considering the small number of subjects and the small increments of dental caries during the short study period. Nonetheless, the observed differences in incremental caries scores between the groups tend to support the favorable results shown by the Swedish studies.

Horowitz, Creighton and McClendon (1971) reported the anticaries effect of weekly rinsing with a 0.2% sodium fluoride solution. Participants in grades 1 and 5 carried out the mouthrinse procedure under the supervision of the classroom teacher. After one year, children in grades 1 and 5 who rinsed with the fluoride solution developed 30 and 28 percent fewer DMF surfaces respectively than children in the control groups. After 20 months, the percentage difference had dropped to 16 percent for grade 1 children, but had increased to 44 percent for children in grade 5.

The use of still another method for self-administration has been reported. In Cheektowaga, New York, children used custom-fitted maxillary and mandibular polyvinyl mouthpieces filled with fluoride gels. One group applied an acidulated phosphate-sodium fluoride gel in a custom-fitted tray for six minutes each school day for two academic years. A second group followed the same application procedure, using a neutral sodium fluoride gel. A third group served as control and received only periodic dental examinations. At the end of 21 months, children who had systematically applied the neutral and acidulated fluoride gels showed outstanding reductions of 75 and 80 percent respectively in incremental DMF surface scores compared with children in the control group. Twenty-three months after the cessation of treatments, the remaining children in the neutral and acidulated fluoride gel groups still retained the advantage of 55 and 63 percent fewer new DMF surfaces than the controls.

Two years after the Cheektowaga study was initiated, Englander and others (1971) began a similar investigation in Charlotte, North Carolina, an optimally fluoridated community. Using custom-fitted trays, test subjects applied the acidulated phosphate-fluoride gel for a period of three minutes, three times a week. Children in the control group received only periodic dental examinations. After 20 months, the treatment regimen had further reduced the already low incremental caries score of children who had consumed fluoridated water all their lives. However, the investigators noted that the extent of added benefit, an average of 0.63 fewer DMF surfaces than control children, was clinically unimpressive.

Although results of the study in Cheektowaga have added much to our knowledge of ultimate decay-preventive benefits that can be attained through self-administered topical fluoride procedures, it is doubtful if a daily application procedure can realistically be considered a feasible public health measure. Experience has taught us that an ideal public health procedure requires little or no conscious action on the part of the individual. For example, in community water fluoridation, the benefits are conferred automatically; no special or deliberate effort is required by the recipient. Before the gel-filled mouthpiece procedure can seriously be considered as having practical public health potential, it must be shown that benefits are conferred when frequency of application is greatly reduced.

Collectively, published data from clinical studies conducted in the Scandinavian countries and more recently in the United States support the efficacy of supervised mouth-rinsing with a weak solution of sodium fluoride. Weekly or fortnightly mouth-rinsing with a 0.2% solution of sodium fluoride has been the most commonly used technic and can be recommended for inclusion in public health programs. The daily use by highly motivated children of a neutral 1.1% sodium fluoride or acidulated phosphate-fluoride gel in custom-fitted trays appears to offer a potent method of caries control. Private practitioners should consider the prescription of this regimen of self-application for such children.

Self-administration of topical fluorides may well provide

the answer to the problems of insufficient professional manpower and excessive costs that currently hinder traditional
topical fluoride programs. With ensuing improvements in
therapeutic agents for caries control and in the technics
of application, self-administration will probably become the
method of choice for topical fluoride application.

TOPICAL FLUORIDE APPLICATION IN AN
OPTIMUM FLUORIDE AREA

Data to support the continued use of topical fluorides in
areas that have begun community fluoridation are rare.
The Council on Dental Therapeutics of the American Dental
Association recommends that "In those communities which
undertake water fluoridation, the topical application of fluorides should be continued for those children whose teeth
were calcified or erupted at the time fluoridation was initiated." The statement is not documented with data to
support the statement.

Muhler (1960) made an evaluation of topically applied
stannous fluoride in a group of children six to 17 years old
in a community that had fluoridated its water supply six
years previously. Results after 30 months of investigation
showed that children in the test group experienced an overall reduction of 54 percent in incremental DMF teeth compared with children in the control group. Although these
results are encouraging, more substantial evidence is
needed on the effectiveness of topical fluoride applications
in relation to age of children at first exposure to fluoridated
water before a substantiated recommendation can be made.
On an empirical basis, it is questionable whether topical
fluoride programs should be continued for more than four
to five years after the start of community fluoridation.

Research is also required to determine if additional
caries protection can be conferred by the topical application of fluoride to the teeth of children who were born and
raised in a fluoride area. No dental benefits were reported
after one year for children who lived in a natural fluoride

area and received topical applications of a 2% sodium fluoride solution. In another one-year study, no appreciable cariostatic effect of sodium fluoride applications in areas of optimum fluoride concentration could be demonstrated. However, both these investigations had few participants and were of short duration. The researchers suggested that additional studies with larger numbers of children should be completed before definite conclusions could be drawn.

Gish and Muhler (1965) tested various combinations of three agents containing stannous fluoride—a prophylaxis paste, a solution, and a dentifrice—in a natural fluoride area and found from 41 to 67 percent fewer DMF surfaces in the test groups than in the control group.

Final results of a three-year study showed that annual, four-minute applications of an 8% stannous fluoride solution to children born and raised in a fluoridated community produced a modest 21 percent reduction in incremental DMF teeth and surfaces. An equally important finding in the investigation was that annual 30-second applications of a 10% stannous fluoride solution produced little, if any, decay-preventive benefits on teeth that had already erupted when the study was started. For teeth that erupted during the first year of study, however, both treatments conferred pronounced and statistically significant benefits.

Because data on the effectiveness of topical fluorides in areas where children have received the full benefits of water fluoridation are limited and equivocal, the procedure cannot currently be recommended for public health programs in those areas.

CONCLUSIONS

Available clinical evidence suggests that the following conclusions can be drawn concerning the effectiveness of various topical fluoride procedures:

The professional application of a 2% solution of sodium fluoride can be recommended as an effective cariostatic procedure; reductions of 30 to 40 percent in the incidence of dental caries have been reported fairly consistently.

A number of studies show topically applied stannous fluoride to be effective in preventing dental caries. However, some recent reports have produced negative results. Because stannous fluoride produces pigmentation of teeth, additional studies should be made in which thorough prophylaxes are given before follow-up examinations to eliminate possible bias in assessing the agent's anticariogenic potential. Another source of error—the reported masking of carious lesions on radiographs as a result of stannous fluoride—should be investigated further.

Ample evidence is available to document the therapeutic value of a professionally applied 1.23% solution of acidulated phosphate-fluoride. Additional clinical trials are required, however, to determine the actual degree of protection conferred. More studies of the agent in gel form are needed.

Because of conflicting findings of studies evaluating the benefits of a stannous fluoride-lava pumice prophylaxis paste, the therapeutic efficacy of this agent is in doubt.

Until greater knowledge about the pharmacologic and therapeutic properties of stannous hexafluorozirconate becomes available, the use of this compound for caries control should not be considered. Published reports of clinical findings to document the efficacy of a new acidulated phosphate fluoride-silicon dioxide prophylaxis paste are lacking, as they are for an acidulated phosphate fluoride-lava pumice paste.

Positive findings of the initial series of clinical studies on the efficacy of annual or semiannual self-applications of a stannous fluoride-zirconium silicate prophylactic paste have, thus far, not been replicated. Results of additional independent studies are needed to determine the anticariogenic effect, if any, from self-application with the new therapeutic paste.

Supervised weekly or fortnightly mouthrinsing with a

0.2% solution of sodium fluoride can no longer be regarded as in the experimental stages. Sufficient data are now available to recommend the self-application technic for use in dental public health programs.

The prescribed daily use of a 1.1% sodium fluoride or acidulated phosphate-fluoride gel in custom-fitted trays should be considered by the private practitioner as a valuable adjunct to caries control in the highly motivated child.

QUESTIONS FOR DISCUSSION

1. If you were in private practice now, what regimen of topical fluoride treatment would you use in your preventive dentistry practice? Why?

2. Conflicting reports on the anticariogenic properties of topically applied stannous fluoride have appeared in the literature. What reasons might be given to explain the divergence in findings?

3. If you had the responsibility for developing a topical fluoride program in a depressed area where there was little professional dental manpower available, what type of program would you initiate?

4. Consider the following set of hypothetical data obtained in a study evaluating two topically applied fluorides in a fluoridated community.

DMF SURFACE INCREMENTS AFTER THREE YEARS FOR
13- TO 15-YEAR-OLD CHILDREN COMPLETING ALL
EXAMINATIONS ACCORDING TO GROUP

Study Group	No. of Children	Mean DMFS Increment	% Difference	95% Confidence Interval*
A (controls)	211	2.50	— —	
B	218	2.20		(-12 to 36)
C	222	1.85		(5 to 47)

* Dubey's method (Dubey, S.D., Lehnhoff, R.W. and Radike, A.W.: 1965. A statistical confidence interval for true percent reduction in caries incidence studies. *J. Dent. Res., 44*:921–923.)

a. What is the percentage difference (reduction) in Group B? In Group C?

b. Are the results significant at 0.05 in Group B? In Group C?

c. What is the mean *annual* increment in the Control Group? Is this value "realistic" for children living in a fluoridated community?

d. How many DMF surfaces were protected from decay among the children in Group C during the three years?

e. If agent C required three hours of a dentist's time during the three years to achieve the benefits shown, is the procedure worthwhile? If the procedure was self-applied?

f. Discuss statistical significance versus practical significance.

FURTHER READING

Bixler, D. and Muhler, J.C.: 1964. Effect on dental caries in children in a non-fluoride area of: combined use of three agents containing stannous fluoride: a prophylactic paste, a solution, and a dentifrice. *J. Am. Dent. Assoc., 68*:792–800.

Englander, H.R., Sherrill, L.T., Miller, B.G., Carlos, J.P., Mellberg, J.R., and Senning, R.S.: 1971. Incremental rates of dental caries after repeated topical sodium fluoride applications in children with lifelong consumption of fluoridated water. *J. Am. Dent. Assoc., 82*:354–358.

Cartwright, H.V., Lindahl, R.L. and Bawden, J.W.: 1968. Clinical findings on the effectiveness of stannous fluoride and acid phosphate fluoride as caries reducing agents in children. *J. Dent. Child., 35*:36–40.

Gish, C.W. and Muhler, J.C.: 1964. Effect on dental caries in children in a natural fluoride area of combined use of three agents containing stannous fluoride: a prophylactic paste, a solution, and a dentifrice. *J. Am. Dent. Assoc., 70*:914–920.

Goaz, P.W., McElwaine, L.P., Biswell, H.A. and White, W.E.: 1963. Effect of daily applications of sodium monofluorophosphate solution on caries rate in children. *J. Dent. Res., 42*:965–972.

Goaz, P.W., McElwaine, L.P., Biswell, H.A. and White, W.E.: 1966. Anticariogenic effect of a sodium monofluorophosphate solution in children after 21 months of use. *J. Dent. Res., 45*:286–290.

Gunz, G.M.: 1971. The effect of self-applied fluoride paste. *J. Public Health Dent., 31*:177–181.

Harris, R.: 1963. Observations on the effect of eight percent stannous fluoride on dental caries in children. *Aust. Dent. J., 8*:335–340.

Heifetz, S.B., Horowitz, H.S. and Driscoll, W.S.: 1970. Two year evaluation of a self-administered procedure for the topical application of acidulated phosphate-fluoride; final report. *J. Public Health Dent., 30*:7–12.

Hennon, D.K. and Muhler, J.C.: 1962. Clinical use of fluorides. *J. Indiana Dent. Assoc., 41*:88–95.

Horowitz, H.S.: 1968. The effect on dental caries of topically applied acidulated phosphate-fluoride: results after one year. *J. Oral Ther., 4*:286–291.

Horowitz, H.S.: 1969. Effect on dental caries of topically applied acidulated phosphate-fluoride: results after two years. *J. Am. Dent. Assoc., 78*:563–572.

Horowitz, H.S.: 1969. Effect of topically applied acidulated phosphate-fluoride on dental caries in Hawaiian school children. IADR Program and Abstracts of Papers, p. 178.

Horowitz, H.S., Creighton, W.E. and McClendon, B.J.: 1971. The effect on human dental caries of weekly oral rinsing with a sodium fluoride mouthwash. *Arch. Oral Biol., 16*:609–616.

Horowitz, H.S. and Lucye, H.S.: 1966. A clinical study of stannous fluoride in a prophylaxis paste and as a solution. *J. Oral Ther., 3*:17–25.

Howell, C.L., Gish, C.W. and Muhler, J.C.: 1955. Effect of topically applied stannous fluoride on dental caries experience in children. *J. Am. Dent. Assoc., 50*:14–17.

Law, F.E., Jeffreys, M.H. and Sheary, H.C.: 1961. Topical applications of fluoride solutions in dental caries control. *Public Health Rep., 76*:287–290.

Muhler, J.C.: 1960. The anticariogenic effectiveness of a single application of stannous fluoride in children residing in an optimal communal fluoride area. II. Results at the end of 30 months. *J. Am. Dent. Assoc., 61*:431–438.

Muhler, J.C.: 1966. Part III: Practical preventive dentistry. *Northwest Dent., 45*:266–270.

Muhler, J.C.: 1968. Mass treatment of children with a stannous fluoride-zirconium silicate self-administered prophylactic paste for partial control of dental caries. *J. Am. Coll. Dent., 35*:45–57.

Muhler, J.C., Kelley, G.E., Stookey, G.K., Lindo, F.I. and Harris, N.O.: 1970. The clinical evaluation of a patient-administered SnF_2-$ZrSiO_4$ prophylactic paste in children. I. Results after one year in the Virgin Islands. *J. Am. Dent. Assoc., 81*:142–145.

Peterson, J.K., Jordan, W.A. and Snyder, J.R.: 1963. Effectiveness of stannous fluoride-silex-silicone prophylaxis paste. Two year report—Moorhead, Minnesota. *Northwest Dent., 42*:276–278.

Peterson, J.K. and Williamson, L.: 1962. Effectiveness of topical application of eight percent stannous fluoride. *Public Health Rep., 77*:39–40.

Torell, P. and Ericsson, Y.: 1965. Two-year clinical tests with different methods of local caries-preventive fluorine application in Swedish schoolchildren. *Acta Odontol. Scand., 23*:287–322.

Wellock, W.D., Maitland, A. and Brudevold, F.: 1965. Caries increments, tooth discoloration, and state of oral hygiene in children given single annual applications of acid phosphate-fluoride and stannous fluoride. *Arch. Oral Biol., 10*:453–460.

Chapter 4

SOCIOLOGICAL, ECONOMICAL AND LEGAL ASPECTS OF FLUORIDATION

S.J. Silverstein, S.J. Wycoff and E. Newbrun

PUBLIC'S ATTITUDES TOWARD FLUORIDATION

In a society which claims to be one of the most health conscious in the world and devotes large amounts of resources towards its preservation, opposition to a scientifically proven method of enhancing health would seem to be contradictory. Yet opposition to fluoridation of public water supplies evokes such outcry that its implementation has been blocked in many communities.

The case for fluoridation is straightforward: it combats the most prevalent of all diseases at little cost and inconvenience and without hazard to health. Analysis of the antifluoridation argument shows that it has three main themes: (1) fluoridation is an experiment which has not been proven in value; (2) fluorides are poisons; (3) treatment by public agencies of the water that everyone must drink is a step in the direction of socialized medicine and an invasion of individual rights.

The effectiveness of fluoridation has been well proven and has been discussed in a previous section. Nevertheless, the evidence is more meaningful to statisticians than to laymen. There are approximately 3 billion unfilled cavities in this country at the present, and neither a problem of this magnitude nor the prospect of reducing this figure makes much impression on the public, which does not regard tooth decay very seriously because it is not deadly nor dramatic.

The most potent of these three arguments is the charge that fluoridating the public water supply infringes on the rights of individuals, "compulsory medication." However, so are smallpox vaccinations and many other modern public health measures. As with smallpox, the individual rights are minor when weighed against the incalculable benefits to our next generation from reduction of disease.

The preceding arguments could be regarded as classic antifluoridation themes. In short, these objections to fluoridation have deep psychological roots. The antifluoridationist has been characterized as opposed to science, authority, or tampering with nature. He also has been characterized as expressing feelings of relative deprivation, alienation, or political conservatism.

Antiscience Attitudes

Some people are suspicious not only of scientific organizations but of the scientists themselves. This stems from the fact that mere literacy, which was the mark of education in the past, simply does not suffice for the age of rapid advances and technological complexities.

In 1953, the Mausners reported a study of 397 voters in Northampton, Massachusetts. Each person interviewed was asked his opinion of pro and antifluoridation statements. At the end of the interview, the person was asked how he expected to vote.

The demographic characteristics were that the antifluoridationists were older and without children under 12 years, people of the lower income brackets and middle or lower-class occupations. Profluoridationists came from younger groups, those in professional, managerial and other white-collar occupations. There was also a significant educational gap between the two groups. A large proportion of the antifluoridationists had failed to finish high school, while most of the profluoridationists finished high school and had college degrees.

These findings strengthen the premise that antiscience attitudes lay behind the antifluoridation reactions:

Almost 95% of those approving fluoridation accept science organization as a reliable source of information on the subject—the antivoter overwhelmingly refused to accept reports of its success or to accept scientific organizations as the best authorities on fluoridation. Many of them felt that public health officials, dentistry, and the chemical industry were in conspiracy to impose the measures on the public.

Attitudes Against Tampering with Nature

Opposition to health legislation covers a wide range of heterogeneity—from groups whose opposition is based on science and reason to those whose objections appear to be based on self-aggrandizement or political consideration. Finally, there are those whose opposition stems from irrational anxieties or lack of understanding. Social changes can be divided into external factors and internal factors. Some external factors involved include threats to power, prestige or economic security of certain groups, the factor of coercion, problems of timing, the attitudes of leadership, and various educational, socioeconomic and cultural factors. The internal factors involved appear to be centered on feelings of "vulnerability" in relation to the sense of bodily wholeness, psychic wholeness, or wholeness of the individuals' "life-space."

Vulnerability has been related to the psycho-analytic theory as "castration anxiety." This essentially means that the basis for most of the irrational anxiety that some health measures arouse in certain individuals is that the measures constitute a threat to their sense of bodily wholeness or their sense of psychic wholeness.

Concept of Relative Deprivation

When one category of people is disadvantaged relative to another, the relatively disadvantaged are likely to compare themselves to the relatively favored. Simmel hypothesized that opposition to fluoridation is likely to be concentrated in categories of people who have a sense of deprivation relative to some reference group.

Economic Deprivation

Survey data indicate that richer people tend to favor fluoridation and poorer people are more likely to oppose it. Also, if educational levels are equalized, this standardization does not eliminate the relation of opinions on fluoridation to income.

Prestige Deprivation

Styles of life or levels of living are indicators associated with common notions of prestige. Of persons interviewed with the highest style and standard of life, 76 percent favored fluoridation; of those rated in the middle, 56 percent favored fluoridation; of those in the lowest group, 38 percent favored fluoridation.

Occupational rank was also used to determine prestige. Highest ranked occupational categories were more favorable to fluoridation than the lowest.

Political Deprivation

This concept generally implies a sense of deprivation of political power relative to others in the community, but not a dissatisfaction with the community government. Respondents with a lower feeling of political efficacy are more opposed to fluoridation.

Rank Disequilibrium

In a pluralistic society people may hold statuses which are widely divergent in terms of their social evaluation. An example of this is, "One can be highly educated, but poor." Simmel found highly educated people with a poor consumption status were found to be hostile to fluoridation. Also, educational level and social life are correlated. Since more highly educated people tend to belong to a greater number of organizations, a highly educated person not belonging to any organization might very well feel especially deprived.

Alienation

Opponents of fluoridation are more likely than proponents to feel that public officials do not really care about what they are thinking and so feel that politics and government are too complicated to understand. It is as if fluoridation symbolizes the buffeting one takes in society where not even the water one drinks is sacred. Also, many opponents have little desire to make the decision themselves, but if they are asked, their answer is *no*. Although "alienation" has been used to explain opposition to fluoridation, this theory may only apply to the staunch antifluoridationists who represent a small segment of the voting population. Sapolsky has proposed an alternative explanation based on voter "confusion," discussed below.

Referenda and Public Opinion

Mr. Louis Harris, of the Harris Opinion Polls, has pointed out that as far as public opinion polls indicate at the outset of any fluoridation campaign the majority of the public, in fact the vast majority—86 percent of the public, have heard of fluoridation and favor it. However, only 54 percent know it prevents caries, 23 percent of the public think it is related to water purification. In spite of this 80-20 lead, two out of three referenda have resulted in water fluoridation being rejected. In other words, from a head start of public opinion in favor, when it gets to the final decision most of the referenda on fluoridation have been lost.

An analysis of fluoridation campaigns suggests that the shift in opinion is due to confusion that develops in the minds of the voters. Only 8 percent of people really believe the poison charge. However, the public information programs, instead of winning over antifluoridationists, are quite likely to create voter anxiety due to exposure to the real and dangerous properties of fluorides if taken in excessive amounts. For a fluoridation referendum to be defeated, the voters do not have to accept completely the antifluoridation arguments; they need only to begin to wonder if there is a risk.

Local Governments

Educated decisions about water fluoridation cannot be made by the use of referenda. This would require that every voter undertake the arduous task of becoming completely informed on a technical issue. Local government officials have the authority to become the decision-makers in the community on health matters, yet frequently they do not act. The question arises, "Why does not local government act and why does fluoridation have trouble?" One reason is that local governments are highly inefficient decision-making structures, whose natural inertia is sufficient to prevent adoption of new measures even when such measures have popular support. Another reason is that there is little political capital to be gained from supporting fluoridation.

Fluoridation enjoys nearly unanimous support from the health professions. The American public approves it and local governments rarely disapprove it. On the other hand, the local government officials are often unwilling to actively support the issue even though the opponents are a "vocal minority." So, one can conclude that the opponents have the power to prevent the adoption of fluoridation only because it takes relatively little power to do so.

ECONOMICS OF FLUORIDATION

In order to appreciate the total impact of water fluoridation in reducing caries, one must also consider the economic gains derived from its use. Two comparisons would be worthwhile: (1) cost of water fluoridation versus fluoride in the other forms and (2) a time-cost comparison of dental treatment in fluoridated areas and nonfluoridated areas.

Cost of Fluoridation

Installation costs for water fluoridation equipment will range between a few hundred dollars and several thousand depending on the size and type of feeder. Operating cost will also vary depending on the equipment and chemical used. Calcium fluoride (fluorspar) is by far the least expensive source of fluoride ion. Sodium silicofluoride is the next cheapest and most widely used. The annual per capita cost of water fluoridation usually runs from 5 to 25 cents. A direct comparison of the annual per capita costs of various fluoride procedures is shown in Table X. Not only is water fluoridation the most economic method but also the most effective.

Chair Time and Cost of Treatment

Since 1945 the water supply in Newburgh, New York, has been fluoridated to a concentration of 1 to 1.2 ppm; the water supply in Kingston, New York, has remained at a fluoride concentration of about 0.05 ppm.

A group of five- and six-year-old children in each city was selected for study. At the time a child was admitted

TABLE X

COST AND EFFICACY OF FLUORIDES IN VARIOUS FORMS

Method	Approximate Yearly Cost per Child (Dollars)	Expected Caries Reduction (percent)	Practicality
Fluoridation of public water supply	0.05–0.25 *	60–65	Excellent
Fluoride tablets and drops	6–11 †	20–40	Poor (for home use) Fair (if given at school)
Fluoride mouthwashes	8	20–50 §	Fair
Fluoride dentifrices	2	15–25	Good
Fluoride topical application	12–24 ††	30–40 §	Good

* Operating cost only, varies with community size
† Consumption depends on age, estimated on retail purchase, as a public health procedure costs would be reduced by group purchase
†† Annual or semiannual
§ Depending on frequency

to the study, all accumulated carious defects were corrected. Thereafter, annual routine incremental care was given.

Costs were computed on a fee-for-service basis, using the New York State Medical fee schedule in 1966. Table XI shows the mean cost needed to provide initial and incremental dental care for Newburgh and Kingston groups. The mean cost in Newburgh remained consistently lower than in Kingston throughout the study. The cost of initial care was 60 percent lower in Newburgh and the incremental care was 50 percent lower.

The mean amount of chair time required to provide both initial and incremental care was 1.6 times greater in Kingston than in Newburgh. This study confirmed that the ingestion of optimally fluoridated water during years of tooth development reduces the initial and progressive caries.

An extremely important effect of a successful fluoridation program is that limited professional manpower time can be conserved so that more patients needing care can be treated. In New Zealand, a survey in a community that had received fluoridated water supplies for some years showed that one dental nurse can provide care for more than 700 children, as compared with 400 children in communities where the water supply is not fluoridated.

TABLE XI

ANNUAL COST OF DENTAL CARE IN A FLUORIDATED AND
NONFLUORIDATED COMMUNITY *

Examination	Age	Mean Cost †	
		Newburgh (fluoridated)	Kingston (nonfluoridated)
Initial	5	$13.86	$33.73
2nd	6	6.85	13.65
3rd	7	8.55	15.70
4th	8	5.44	13.41
5th	9	8.62	13.30
6th	10	5.18	11.23

* Adjusted for race
† Cost is corrective care, excluding costs of examination, prophylaxis and radiographs

FLUORIDATION AND THE LAW

Opponents to fluoridation have raised three fundamental constitutional questions—two under the fourteenth amendment* and one under the first amendment.† In the infringement of individual liberty cases, 30 courts have decided that due process was not violated. The claim that equal protection of the laws was not afforded under programs alleged to be discriminatory because they were primarily for children has been rejected as without merit as have the claims of infringement on religious freedom.

Lack of Municipal Authority

The basic argument on the question of municipal authority to fluoridate is that the municipality *lacks* such authority because it is not expressly granted by statute or municipal charter and because it is not reasonable to imply such authority from general grant of "police powers" delegated to a municipality by the legislature.

Here, a *minority* of trial courts have agreed that the authority to fluoridate public water supplies could not reasonably be taken to flow from a general police power granted to municipalities; the appellate courts have unanimously decided that although the statutes do not specifically authorize fluoridation, they do authorize municipalities to pass health measures, and that fluoridation is a health measure even though it is not directed at a contagious disease. Cities have implied authority to pass fluoridation ordinances as a valid exercise of the police power.

---

* Amendment XIV: Citizenship, Representation and Payment of Public Debt. . . . No state shall make or enforce any law which shall abridge the privileges or immunities of citizens of the United States; nor shall any state deprive any person of life, liberty or prosperity without due process of law; nor deny to any person within its jurisdiction the equal protection of the laws.

† Amendment I: Restrictions on Powers of Congress. Congress shall make no law respecting an establishment of religion, or prohibiting the free exercise thereof. . . .

Abuse of Municipal Authority

Conceding the existence of municipal authority to promote and preserve public health and recognizing that the prevention of oral disease is within the purview of public health, the opponents of fluoridation have, nonetheless, attacked fluoridation ordinances as unconstitutional. In order to be successful, this argument must establish that fluoridation is an *unreasonable* and arbitrary exercise of police power, or that it violates rights specifically granted by state and federal constitutions.

The exercise of the police power must be reasonable. An *unreasonable* exercise amounts to a "taking" of life, liberty or property without due process of law or a violation of the "privileges and immunities" or "equal protection" guaranteed by the fourteenth amendment.

The opponents of fluoridation have contended that fluoridation is unreasonable because it is

1. Unnecessary
2. Wasteful
3. Unsafe
4. Class legislation (discriminatory legislation)
5. Breach of contract between the municipality and its water consumers
6. An illegal use of public funds
7. A nuisance
8. Compulsory medication and thereby violates certain fundamental liberties
9. An alternative method available to accomplish whatever benefit might be ascribed to fluoridation.

Violation of Religious Freedom

Perhaps the most difficult and least adequately answered objection to fluoridation is the argument that an ordinance providing for fluoridation forecloses full choice on the part of the consumer and, in effect, requires him to consume public water which contains additives repugnant to his religious convictions and violates the first amendment (religious freedom).

Religious freedom has received attention in recent years, but judicial opinion has not been unamimous on either the extent of religious guarantees or the essential nature of religious guarantees or the essential nature of religious liberty.

A point raised by the court tends to support the proponents' position. Fluorides exist naturally in the public waters of many communities, sometimes in quantities in excess of the optimum amount. The court observed that the city in such circumstances would not be required to remove the natural fluoride from the supply.

Violation of Specific Statutes

Plaintiffs' pleadings frequently have included an allegation that the fluoridation ordinance being attacked violates a specific state statute. The statutes usually involved have been pure food and drug acts and statutes forbidding the unauthorized practice of medicine, dentistry or pharmacy.

Pure Food Acts. Opponents assert that fluoridation violates the following acts:

1. An adulteration of food
2. Violation of a "poisons" statute
3. Violation of statutes forbidding the adulteration of nonalcoholic beverages.

Several courts have upheld proponents' answers to the effect that the addition of 1 ppm of fluoride, being a measure approved by medical and public health authorities, does not amount to adulteration within the meaning of the prohibitory statutes involved.

In another case, it was held that "the purpose of the statute is to regulate and restrict the retail sale of poisons as such," and that the addition of 1 ppm fluoride to the water supply "cannot under any reasonable theory be held to be a sale or retail of fluoride within the meaning of the

. . . [statute]." The court further observed that the same prohibitory statute listed nicotine.

State Laws Requiring Fluoridation

Fluoridation decision-making is moving from the local to the state level. This allows educational efforts to be narrowed down to a small audience—the legislators.

The following states have passed laws requiring fluoridation of domestic water supplies:

1. Connecticut: Implemented in 1965 for all cities with populations exceeding 20,000. The action was initiated as a regulation of the State Health Department.

2. Minnesota: Enacted in 1967 this law requires fluoridation of all municipal water supplies by 1970.

3. Illinois: A 1967 law applying to all water supplies.

4. Delaware: In 1968, Delaware enacted a law authorizing the State Board of Health to order fluoridation.

5. Michigan: In 1968, Michigan enacted the first law that included a provision for a referendum. The law requires all communities to take action on fluoridation within five years; exemption is allowed by local ordinance or referendum.

6. South Dakota: Enacted in 1969, the law applies to all communities of 500 or more. A bill to repeal the law was rejected in the lower House of the Legislature, but a bill to require a statewide referendum is pending.

7. Ohio: In 1970, a law was enacted that requires fluoridation of all water supplies serving 5,000 or more persons. The State Health Department will reimburse the community for the purchase and installation of equipment. It also provided that a referendum petition could be filed during a 120-day period after the law went into effect.

The Case of California

California ranks close to the bottom in a list of States ranked according to the number of persons receiving fluoride in their water supply. Several factors have combined to produce this result:

1. California has a 60-year tradition of using referenda and has depended on local referenda to decide local fluoridation issues.

2. The fluoridation issue has proven most difficult to settle on its merits due to scare campaigns.

3. State and local political leaders have tended to shun involvement.

4. At the local level, water is often supplied not by the cities but by agencies and districts.

How Can California Improve Its Fluoridation Standing?

1. The State Board of Public Health could make a determination that public health and welfare require the maintenance of adequate fluoride content in all public water supply systems.

2. The legislature could consider enacting a law specifically declaring fluoride a matter of statewide policy.

3. The governor could appoint a special state commission to study dental health and fluoridation and to formulate recommendations.

4. Local elected officials could be urged to study fluoridation and adopt public positions on the issue.

5. Community leaders and participants in antipoverty programs could assist low-income citizens to understand the problems.

QUESTIONS FOR DISCUSSION

1. If unlimited funds are available how would you go about planning a campaign to alter public opinion in favor of fluoridation?

2. Within the next five to seven years a national health insurance which will cover dental care may be in effect. How would fluoridation affect the cost of this insurance program?

3. Why will the Supreme Court not rule on the constitutionality of fluoridation?

4. An individual accepts the epidemiological findings that water fluoridation reduces caries. He is not concerned with the "poison" charge. However, he believes that there is a grave danger that if the government is allowed to add fluoride to drinking water, if could also add other chemicals or drugs, i.e. "mass medication." How would you answer him?

5. Many people who are involved in the ecology movement believe that fluoride which is not used by the body passes into the waste water and contributes to the contamination of the environment. How would you answer them?

FURTHER READING

Ast, D.B., Cons, N.C., Pollard, S.F. and Garfinkel, J.: 1970. Time and cost factors to provide regular, periodic dental care for children in a fluoridated and nonfluoridated area: final report. *J. Am. Dent. Assoc., 80:* 770–776.

Clark, R.E. and Sophy, M.M.: 1967. Fluoridation in the courts and the opposition. *Wayne Law Review, 13:*338.

Crain, R.L., Katz, E. and Rosenthal, D.B.: 1969. *The Politics of Community Conflict: the Fluoridation Decision.* Indianapolis, Bobbs-Merrill.

Gamson, W.A. and Irons, P.H.: 1961. Community characteristics and fluoridation outcome. *J. Social Issues, 17:*66–74.

Linn, E.L.: Spring 1969. Effect of community leaders and organizations on public attitudes toward fluoridation. *J. Public Health Dent., 29:*108–17.

Mausner, B. and Mausner, J.: 1955. A study of the anti-scientific attitude; with biographical sketch of the authors. *Sci. Am., 192:*35–39.

Nathan, H. and Scott, S.: 1966. Fluoridation in California: An unresolved public policy issue. *Bull. Inst. Gov. Stud.,* vol. 7, no. 5.

Sapolsky, H.M.: 1968. Science, voters and the fluoridation controversy. *Science, 162:*427–433.

Simmel, A.: 1961. A signpost for research on fluoridation conflicts: the concept of relative deprivation. *J. Social Issues, 17:*26–36.

Strong, G.A.: 1967. Liberty, religion and fluoridation. *Santa Clara Lawyer, 8:*37–58.

Chapter 5

THE MECHANISM OF THE ANTICARIES ACTION OF FLUORIDE ION

H.M. Myers

Two properties of the fluoride ion (F⁻) dominate any consideration of its anticaries action. The first of these is its similarity to the hydroxyl ion (OH⁻). Both ions have a primary hydration number of 5 and ionic radii of very similar dimensions: 1.29 Å for F⁻ and 1.33 Å for OH⁻. By way of comparison, the closest halogen, chloride, has a primary hydration number of 2 and radius of 1.88 Å.

The second property of fluoride ion deserving attention is its ability to inhibit enzyme action. Here its role is complex and its action is usually classified according to the metal ion requirement shown by the enzyme. The mechanisms for each of these groups of enzymes is thought to be different. Significant inactivation of enzymes by fluoride generally occurs in the region 10^{-4} to 10^{-3} M. Some enzymatic inhibition, however, has been reported at 5×10^{-5} M, which corresponds to 1 ppm.

SYSTEMIC FLUORIDE AND THE APATITE CRYSTAL

The effect of fluoride ions on the apatite lattice has been studied by both qualitative and quantitative x-ray diffraction methods.

The poor resolution given by the minute crystals of apatite with x-rays makes it difficult to analyze precisely the effect of fluoride on the apatite lattice. Improved resolution of the diffraction peaks can be obtained by heating the samples. This observation, long known in crystallography, is due to several considerations. Heating, at the temperatures used, causes increased crystallite size, and this in turn gives a larger number of atomic diffraction planes with which the x-ray beam can interact. The result is an improved diffraction pattern with sharper, more well-defined peaks. The width of the diffraction peaks is narrowed, and the degree of overlap of the several peaks is lessened. The same effect may be observed when strain due to imperfections in the crystals is eliminated (as also would occur with heating). Thus, it is possible to assess the degree of crystallinity of apatites by comparing samples with a series of idealized diffraction curves. The closer to the ideal of sharp solitary peaks the specimen yields, the higher is the degree of crystallinity. Crystallinity in this sense refers to the combined effects of (1) increased crystal size and (2) lack of strain in the lattice on the shape and sharpness of the diffraction peaks. A comparative method such as this is empirical in that it measures deviations from a standardized composite curve derived only partially from theoretical considerations. Using this method, fluoride ion has been shown to improve the crystallinity of apatite in bones and teeth.

If all the mineral in calcified tissue were in the form of hydroxyapatite, it should be possible to predict the height and size of the diffraction peaks. When this is done, the observed peak size is always less than predicted. This may be interpreted as being due to the fact that some portion of the mineral is amorphous and gives no x-ray diffraction pattern. The relative amount of such mineral can be estimated from the difference between the observed peak size and the predicted theoretical values. This observed difference has been attributed to the presence of "amorphous calcium phosphate." It has been demonstrated that fluoride ion promotes the conversion of amorphous calcium phosphate into hydroxyapatite. This is one way in which fluoride can be said to increase the crystallinity of apatite.

More quantitative methods of studying the influence of fluoride on apatite structure have come from the use of neutron diffraction along with high precision x-ray diffraction methods. Neutron diffraction is the ideal method of studying the position of hydrogen atoms in crystals. X-rays have an insignificant degree of interaction with hydrogens, but this is not true of neutrons which are significantly stopped by this smallest of the atoms. Studies with neutron diffraction have located the positions of the hydrogens of the hydroxyl ions in the apatite lattice. This in turn has given rise to an atomic interpretation of the role of fluoride in apatite structure which is known as the "void theory." This theory is consistent with the idea that fluoride ions improve the crystallinity of apatite by eliminating voids in the crystal structure, which when present contribute to strain and give poorer x-ray diffraction patterns. The data on which this theory is based are more quantitative than the empirical comparisons used to assess degree of crystallinity directly. Exact positions of the atoms in apatite are determined, and from these atomic dimensions the role of fluoride is postulated.

The appearance of fluoride ion in bone and tooth mineral (hydroxyapatite) is readily explained by the similarity of hydroxyl and fluoride ions. The ready replacement of hydroxyl ions by fluoride ions is usually thought to imply no structural change in the crystal lattice. Actually, even for this obviously isomorphous replacement there occurs a slight shortening of the *a* axis of hydroxyapatite. Fluoride can fit perfectly in the center of the triangular arrangement of calcium ions present in the apatite structure (Fig. 8). Fluoride ions, thus, lie in the same plane as calciums of that triangle. Hydroxyl ions, on the other hand, are displaced 0.3 Å to either side of that plane and are so oriented that their hydrogens are directed away from the plane. A line drawn through the hydrogen and oxygen of the hydroxyl group is the *c* axis and would be perpendicular to the plane of the calcium triangles. Fluoride ions, when present, lie at a point where the line exactly crosses the plane formed by the three calcium ions.

In order to maintain symmetry, hydroxyl ions must be

located on one side of the plane as often as on the other. If the hydroxyl ion is randomly arranged with respect to the side of the plane it occupies, there would be reversal points due to the orientation of hydroxyl groups in the apatite lattice. These reversal points are caused by hydroxyl ions pointing their hydrogens either away from or toward one another. Neutron diffraction measurements show that two adjacent calcium planes could not have two hydroxyl ions between them if their hydrogens were oriented toward each other. Where such orientation of hydroxyl groups occurs (one pointing its hydrogen down from upper triangle and one pointing up from the lower), steric interference would occur. A structure of this type could not accommodate both hydroxyls, and one of the hydroxyl ions would of necessity be deleted, creating a void. Voids are not uncommon in crystals, but their presence leads to greater chemical reactivity, such as increased solubility. If a fluoride ion were to replace the missing hydroxyl ion, it would eliminate the void by occupying it. Recall that it does not occupy the exact same spot as the hydroxyl ion. This would stabilize the crystal structure by providing additional and significantly stronger hydrogen bonds at sites which previously had none. Such increased stability would be reflected in a decreased mobility of the residual ions. This latter property is understandably related to the ease with which acids (H^+ ions) can disrupt apatite structure.

The number of reversal points in which fluoride ions can replace missing hydroxyl ions is unknown, but it clearly cannot be large or there would be no tendency for the hydroxyapatites to be as stable as they are in water. The need for only a small number of fluoride ions to replace missing hydroxyl ions is what makes this theory of fluoride ion action so attractive.

The amount of fluoride needed to replace all the hydroxyls of hydroxyapatite is 2 per unit cell. If this were to occur the amount of fluoride would be 38,000 ppm. Enamel formed under the influence of 1 ppm fluoride in drinking water has about 1000 to 2000 ppm in its outermost surface. Clearly, the conversion of hydroxy to fluorapatite is minimal under these conditions (3% to 5%) and reference to the physical properties of fluorapatite to explain the action of fluoride ion on enamel is inappropriate. However, void replacement would require only a small increment of fluoride ion to produce a profound effect on the physical properties of the partially substituted hydroxyapatite.

More direct experimental support for the void replacement concept comes from the technique of nuclear magnetic resonance. With this physical method the environments of fluoride ions in apatite can be compared. Fluoride ions can be grouped according to the similarity of their atomic surroundings. In apatites with small amounts of fluoride (8%) two distinct patterns of fluoride environments can be shown. The first of these represents fluoride ions which have two equally close hydrogen atoms 2.13 Å away, 180 degrees apart. This can be represented by OHFHO. A second group of fluoride ions has one hydrogen atom 2.13 Å away but the other is 180 degrees away at a distance of 4.75 Å. This arrangement can be represented by OHFOH. The "OHFHO" pattern reflects the situation where a hydroxyl ion is replaced by a fluoride ion and the neighboring hydroxyl ions are oriented with their hydrogens pointing toward the fluoride ion. The "OHFOH" pattern refers to a fluoride-filled void in which the closer hydrogen is oriented toward the fluoride and the distant one away from it. Figure 8 presents a schematic drawing of this arrangement.

The fact that two distinct environments for fluoride in apatite have been found is strong evidence that reversal points actually occur within a single column of calcium triangles. The fact that two hydroxyls cannot be accommodated spatially in two adjacent triangles if their hydrogens point toward one another does not of itself require that voids exist. It is possible that all the hydroxyls in a given column of calcium triangles could be oriented in the same direction. The averaging out of their positions could be produced if

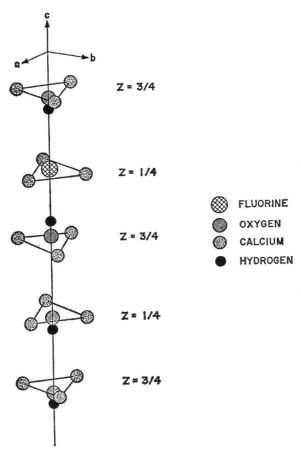

Figure 8. Perspective drawing of calcium triangle arrangement indicates the two possible hydroxyl ion positions. A void (second triangle from the top) has been replaced by a fluoride ion. The arrangement of the three upper triangles can be represented by OHFHO. If the hydroxyl ion in the third triangle were below the plane with its hydrogen pointing down, the representation would be OHFOH. The vectors *a, b* and *c* are crystal axes. The *z* values and fractions represent the fractional distance along the *c* axis of the unit cell. Portions of three unit cells are shown. The complete unit cell begins midway between the first and second triangles and ends between the third and fourth. (Courtesy Professor Young [1966] *Arch. Oral Biol.*)

alternating columns had opposite orientations of their hydroxyl groups—each column of calcium triangles would have either the up or down direction of its hydroxyl groups. All that would be required to give the observed symmetry for the hydroxyl positions would be an equal number of up and down columns. There would be no requirement for missing hydroxyls if this were the case. However, a fluoride ion which replaced such a hydroxyl ion would always have one neighboring hydroxyl with its hydrogen close to it (2.13 Å) and the hydroxyl on the opposite side with its hydrogen pointing away from it (4.75Å). Regardless of the overall orientation of the hydroxyls of any column, there would always be only *one* environment—OHFOH for the fluoride. Thus, reversal points must be present within a column of hydroxyls if both OHFOH and OHFHO are found.

Since the presence of reversal points implies voids and since fluoride ions can fit in those voids while hydroxyls cannot, a molecular interpretation of the stabilizing- and crystallinity-increasing effect of fluoride can be formulated.

It is possible, therefore, to explain the systemic action of fluoride on caries as being due to a stabilization of the apatite lattice. Such stabilization is a result of hydroxyapatite having inherent voids due to missing hydroxyl groups. Fluoride ions fill the voids and add their hydrogen-bonding tendency to the forces which hold the crystal together.

ACTION OF FLUORIDE TOPICALLY

The use of topical applications of fluoride to reduce dental decay involves much higher concentrations of fluoride than does water fluoridation. A 2% solution of NaF has about 9000 mg of fluoride per liter, compared to a liter of water with 1 ppm fluoride which has 1 mg of fluoride.

There is some doubt that a permanent fluoride ion increase in enamel always occurs after topical application. Recent studies using topical solutions with 12,000 mg/liter of fluoride have shown no significant increase in fluoride content of enamel. Levels of 1000 to 1500 ppm before application returned to the same level five to eight weeks after the application. If a brief one-minute etching of the enamel with phosphoric acid is employed prior to the use of topical fluoride, substantial increases can be detected over the same period. Final values of up to 5000 ppm can be shown to be present. Use of fluoride in acid media of pH 3 to 4 gives maximal uptake. The effect of acid pH on fluoride uptake is related to the increased mobility of hydroxyl ions in the lattice. This is equivalent to saying that fluoride ions and hydroxyl ions can exchange more readily at acid pH. Topical fluoride following acid treatment may allow fluoride ions to replace voids formed by the acid. The increase in fluoride is of such magnitude, however, as to suggest that more than just hydroxyl void replacement is occurring. Additional surface films of such protective insoluble salts as CaF_2 are also likely involved.

Although even larger initial uptakes of fluoride ion than indicated above can occur with topical treatment, 90 percent is readily removed by washing. The remaining portion has been identified by x-ray diffraction to be in the form of both CaF_2 and fluorapatite. Good evidence exists for the presence of topically incorporated fluoride ion at a depth of 50μ from the surface.

Stannous fluoride apparently produces both CaF_2 and tin-fluoride-phosphate salt, both of which are highly insoluble. The products of reaction between SnF_2 and enamel include an uncertain crystal type thought to be $Sn_3F_3PO_4$. Stannous ions may promote stability of the new surface phase by virtue of their high polarizability. Surface energy and therefore resistance to solvents is lowered by the presence of a polarizable cation. Polarizability refers to the distortion of the electron cloud of an ion in the presence of unevenly distributed positive charges, such as occurs at a crystal surface. High degrees of such distortion tend to spread out the negative charge of the electron cloud and to reduce the imbalance of surface charges. This reduces the energy necessary to hold a surface together and therefore stabilizes the surface.

There is indirect evidence from kinetic analysis of the rate of dissolution of hydroxyapatite that CaF_2 forms on the surface due to the release and reprecipitation of calcium from the apatite in the presence of high levels of fluoride. A layer of fluorapatite slowly builds up between the hydroxyapatite and the CaF_2, and this layer is responsible for some of the resistance to acid dissolution (and caries) produced by topical fluorides.

Topical sodium fluoride has long been known to react at the surface of hydroxyapatite to produce CaF_2 and cause the release of inorganic phosphate. The release of phosphate is increased at low pH. In effect, topical NaF slightly dissolves the surface of apatite and causes reprecipitation of the calcium as CaF_2. The phosphate is lost in solution. The currently more popular topical agents all give rise to CaF_2 but appear to have an additional feature of retarding the loss of phosphate.

Stannous fluoride as mentioned earlier is believed to form an insoluble complex salt of fluoride phosphate and tin in addition to CaF_2. Acidulated phosphofluoride provides the acid medium to promote fluoride uptake but also provides a source of phosphate ions to counteract the tendency for this ion to escape from the crystal surface into the ambient solution. A portion of this retardation of phosphate loss is likely due to fluorapatite formation.

Monofluorophosphate is rapidly hydrolyzed into fluoride and phosphate at the enamel surface. The phosphate produced may also serve to counteract the tendency of apatite to lose this ion during the CaF_2 reaction.

The hydrolysis of monofluorophosphate is apparently catalyzed only by hydroxyapatite or enamel surfaces. Fluorapatite, calcium oxalate or zinc phosphate have no effect on the fluorophosphate ion. The release of fluoride ion by fluorophosphate is very likely the basis of its anticaries action. The hydrolysis can also be catalyzed by the enzyme acid phosphatase which has been found in salivary sediment. It presumably is present also in dental plaque, and the splitting of this complex fluoride ion by plaque could play a role in caries prevention. This concept is reinforced by the fact that intact enamel does not incorporate as much fluoride ion directly from monofluorophosphate as it does from other topical preparations. The effectiveness of MFP preparations may therefore be due to the release of fluoride ion from fluorophosphate by dental plaque as the initial step in providing fluoride ion. Low pH is known also to favor the hydrolysis.

A topical effect of fluoride ion may be involved in the marginal sealing effect of certain dental restorations. Silicate powders are manufactured with the use of a flux containing considerable fluoride. Silicate cements can reduce the solubility of enamel adjacent to them by about 20 percent. The effect is correlated with an increased fluoride uptake greater than that produced by 2% NaF. Most of the relative infrequency of secondary caries associated with silicates may be related to this effect. Cements which have no fluoride content, such as zinc phosphates, do not have the solubility-reducing effect.

When 1.5% SnF_2 was incorporated into amalgam alloy, the enamel adjacent to the filling was less soluble in acid after a few days of contact with the filling. The fluoride content of this less soluble enamel was increased by about 33 percent. Unfortunately, only phosphate release was measured and, as indicated above, this is not likely to be a simple straightforward measure of enamel solubility after treatment with SnF_2. Controls with only stannous ions such as $SnCl_2$ were not used.

ENZYME INHIBITION BY FLUORIDE

The demonstration that fluoride is present both in the surface of enamel and in dental plaque in relatively higher concentrations than elsewhere has revived interest in the enzyme-inhibiting properties of this ion. The low level of fluoride ion in the extracellular fluids (0.15 ppm) generally precludes any enzyme inhibition, but higher levels in enamel and plaque may release sufficient fluoride to allow an inhibitory effect.

It will be recalled at this point that the outermost enamel has been shown to have fluoride levels approaching 1500 ppm; this can be temporarily increased by topical treatment or fluoride-containing dentifrices. The subsequent loss of such fluoride increments in itself indicates that the ion is available to solutions bathing the teeth.

Lactic acid formation by *Lactobacillus casei* has been shown to be inhibited 32 percent when fluorosed intact enamel was incubated with the organism. Topical treatment with NaF and SnF_2 also produces reduced lactate yields of the same order of magnitude. Raising the concentration of fluoride and lowering the pH of the solutions, which should increase the inhibitory action, has only a variable and erratic effect on lactate formation. Thus, the importance of fluoride in enamel as a glycolysis inhibitor remains uncertain. If is not clear that the degrees of inhibition observed will be significant in the pathogenesis of caries.

Only the phosphoglyceromutase- and enolase-catalyzed reactions are inhibited significantly (more than 50%) by 38 ppm of various fluoride-containing salts. The most effective source of fluoride ion in this regard is NaF and an amine hydrofluoride. Fluosilicate has a wide spectrum of inhibition, but its action is less pronounced.

The long chain protonated amines (aliphatic amines with a positively charged nitrogen) are capable of binding to the surface of enamel as well and may be effective by retarding the dissolution rate. Decreasing solubility of enamel correlates well with increasing carbon chain length in the range between 10 and 16 carbons.

Levels of fluoride which are definitely inhibitory to enzymes usually are about 30 ppm. Dental plaque and calculus may contain somewhat lower levels (14 to 19 ppm), but it is doubtful that all of this fluoride can be mobilized as ions. Fluoride in dental plaque appears to be only about 10 percent ionic, which would give fluoride ion levels of 1 to 2 ppm. The latter apparently is just able to inhibit enolase *in vitro*.

In vitro inhibition of enzymes, especially enolase, can only be related to *in vivo* effects with considerable caution. Fluoride inhibition of this enzyme requires both magnesium ions and inorganic phosphate. Competition for the phosphate by other reactions can reduce inhibitory action of fluoride to insignificant levels.

Amine fluorides, but not simple inorganic fluorides, can block the formation of extracellular deposits by *Streptococcus mutans in vitro*. This activity may also be due to the surface active properties of amine fluorides as well as the fluoride ion. Fluoride does not inhibit the glucosyltransferase involved in bacterial extracellular polysaccharide synthesis. In addition, no difference in the dry deposit weight of ten-day-old calculus has been found in individuals using fluoride-free and fluoride-containing dentifrices. This is true even though the fluoride content varied fivefold—from 154 ppm in the nonfluoride group to 702 in the fluoride group.

Bacterial intracellular polysaccharide synthesis by *Streptococcus mitis* is reduced in amount if the organism is exposed to 10 ppm of fluoride or more. The effect, however, may be due to impaired uptake of glucose rather than enzyme inhibition of the polysaccharide-synthesizing steps. Acid formation falls parallel to polysaccharide formation immediately after introducing fluoride to the respiring cells. In addition, fluoride added externally to cells is more effective than fluoride taken up by cells. Even if one could demonstrate direct inhibition of isolated enzymes from such cells, the action of fluoride could still be due to interference with substrate uptake, leading to both reduced synthesis of polysaccharide and glycolysis of glucose.

It is important to realize that both the inhibition of glycolysis and the apatite-strengthening effect are mutually compatible. The relatively small amount of fluoride found in enamel would appear to stabilize the apatite lattice. At the same time, enamel can provide fluoride for plaque and calculus. This in turn could have a small effect on the rate of acid formation. Both these effects of fluoride could be involved in caries inhibition *in vivo*.

QUESTIONS FOR DISCUSSION

1. Would you expect topical and systemic administration of fluoride to have additive effects? Should topical fluorides and fluoride-containing dentifrices be recommended by dentists in areas where water fluoridation is practiced?

2. How would you answer the charge that fluoride ion is an enzyme poison and should not be used in preventive measures such as water fluoridation?

3. What value can you assign to a technique that incorporates more fluoride into a developing tooth? Would you take the same position about a technique which claimed to add more fluoride to the enamel surface after topical use?

4. Biopsy of surface enamel in a nonfluoride area revealed 500 ppm of fluoride. Assuming enamel to be only apatite $[Ca_{10}(PO_4)_6(OH)_2]$, to what extent (%) have the hydroxyl groups been replaced by fluoride?

$$\text{Atomic weights: } Ca = 40$$
$$P = 31$$
$$H = 1$$
$$O = 16$$
$$F = 19$$

FURTHER READING

Baud, C.A. and Bang, S.: 1970. Electron probe and X-ray diffraction microanalyses of human dental enamel treated in vitro by fluoride solution. *Caries Res., 4*:1–13.

Briner, W.W. and Francis, M.D.: 1962. The effect of enamel fluoride on acid production by *Lactobacillus casei. Arch. Oral Biol., 7*:541–50.

Brudevold, F., Aasenden, R., McCann, H.G., III and McCann, H.G.: 1969. Use of an enamel biopsy method for determination of in vivo uptake of fluoride from topical treatments. *Caries Res., 3*:119–33.

Capozzi, L., Brunetti, P., Negri, P.L. and Migliorini, E.: 1967. Enzymatic mechanism of some fluorine compounds. *Caries Res., 1*:69–77.

Grön, P., Brudevold, F. and Aasenden, R.: 1971. Monofluorophosphate interaction with hydroxyapatite and intact enamel. *Caries Res., 5*:202–14.

Jerman, A.C.: 1970. Silver amalgam restorative material with SnF_2. *J. Am. Dent. Assoc., 80*:787–91.

Norman, R.D., Phillips, R.W. and Swartz, M.L.: 1960. Fluoride uptake by enamel from certain dental materials. *J. Dent. Res., 39*:11–16.

Omachi, A., Deuticke, B. and Gerlach, E.: 1966. Fluoride inhibition of erythrocyte metabolism as a function of cellular inorganic phosphate *Biochim. Biophys. Acta, 124*:421–4.

Phillips, R.W. and Swartz, M.L.: 1957. Effect of certain restorative mate rials on solubility of enamel. *J. Am. Dent. Assoc., 54*:623–36.

Posner, A.S.: 1969. Crystal chemistry of bone mineral. *Physiol. Rev., 49*: 760–92.

Schroeder, H.E.: 1969. *Formation and Inhibition of Dental Calculus*. Berne, Hans Huber, pp. 91–93.

Singer, L., Jarvey, B.A., Venkateswarlu, P. and Armstrong, W.D.: 1967. Fluoride in plaque. *J. Dent. Res., 49*:455.

Van der Lugt, W., Knottnerus, D.I.M. and Young, R. A.: 1970. NMR determination of fluorine positions in mineral hydroxyapatite. *Caries Res., 4*:89–95.

Wiseman, A.: 1970. Effect of inorganic fluoride on enzymes. In F.A. Smith (Ed.): *Handbook of Exp. Pharmacol.*, part 2. Berlin, Springer Verlag, pp. 48–97.

Chapter 6

FLUORIDE METABOLISM

I. Zipkin

INTRODUCTION

Fluoride, chiefly as fluorspar or fluorite (CaF_2), fluorapatite ($Ca_{10}[PO_4]_6F_2$), or cryolite (Na_3AlF_6) is the thirteenth most abundant element in the earth's crust and exists in higher concentration than chlorine, sulfur, carbon, copper or nitrogen. Oxygen is the most abundant at 46.4 percent.

Fluoride is the most chemically reactive of all the anions or negatively charged ions. It does not occur as the element, except in a violet-blue-colored fluorspar, which when powdered gives a smell of fluorine.

Fluoride or fluorine is derived from the Latin *fluore*, to flow, since it was used as a flux, that is, to promote the fusion of certain metal ores such as aluminum oxide.

In 1670, a Nüremberg artist, Schwanhard, appeared to be the first to etch glass from vapors generated by the action of sulfuric acid on fluorspar. This was probably an empirical finding. In 1771, Scheele, a Swedish apothecary, produced hydrogen fluoride in aqueous solution; Gay-Lussac of gas-law fame described the corrosive action of the acid on skin in 1809. Elemental fluorine, a greenish-yellow gas with a sharp irritating odor, was first isolated by Moissan in 1886.

In 1803, Dominico Morichini, an Italian chemist, showed fluoride to be present in a fossil elephant tooth. Along with Gay-Lussac, he showed fluoride to be present in fresh human and animal teeth as well. About 1846, George Wilson, a Scottish chemist, showed fluoride to be widespread in fresh and sea water, in vegetables, in blood and milk, and thus to be ubiquitously distributed. In 1867, the first animal experiments seem to have been made by Rabuteau, followed by Tappeiner, Schulz and Brandl about 1890.

Fluorine exists in organic combination in insulating materials such as tygon, in refrigerant gases such as freon, in steroids such as 9-α-fluorohydrocortisone and in anesthetics such as methoxyflurane and halothane. The metabolism of these compounds to produce fluoride ion through enzymatic processes is unknown and needs to be investigated. Recent evidence indicates, for example, that methoxyflurane may liberate fluoride ion with comparative ease in the human.

Although fluoride is classed with the halogens, it does not behave like one from a number of viewpoints. Chemically, silver fluoride is soluble in water, whereas the other silver halides are insoluble. More importantly, however, fluoride does not behave physiologically like the other halogens. The ion is rapidly deposited in bone whereas chloride, bromide and iodide are present in only trace amounts. In addition, the thyroid gland, which accumulates iodide easily, does not incorporate fluoride in appreciable amounts. Finally, the kidney clears fluoride with much greater rapidity than it does the other halogens. Thus, fluoride is a very unusual ion with an ubiquitous distribution in nature and with physiological properties differentiating it from the other halogens. In addition, it may also be described as being a highly emotional element, in view of the extensive controversies it has stirred up in many communities considering the fluoridation of municipal water supplies for the partial control of dental caries.

ABSORPTION

Absorption may be defined as transport of materials across the lumen of the gastrointestinal tract upon ingestion, to be taken up by the capillaries and distributed throughout the body for utilization.

In balance studies, the amount of the material ingested as well as that excreted in the urine and feces is measured in a 24-hour period. Unless the expired air (insensible perspiration) and the skin (sensible perspiration) represent appreciable avenues of loss, they are usually disregarded. Thus, the difference between the amounts ingested and that excreted in the feces represents what has been absorbed, since fecal excretion represents unused material, i.e. passed on through the gastrointestinal tract and voided. Some of the absorbed material (that passed through the gastrointestinal membranes eventually to the general circulation) is deposited in the body and the remainder is excreted in the urine. Thus, amount ingested minus that excreted (amount excreted in urine plus amount excreted in feces) equals amount deposited in the body. In this way, balances can be determined for calcium, phosphorus, magnesium, nitrogen or fluoride, as well as for others.

Mechanism and Site of Absorption

Fluoride appears to be absorbed, that is, passes through the walls of the gastrointestinal tract to blood and eventually into other body fluids and tissues by rather direct and simple diffusion, rather than requiring energy or enzymatic processes for transport.

Absorption seems to take place from various portions of the gastrointestinal tract, that is the stomach and the small intestine. Both *in vitro* and *in vivo* experiments have been done to show that absorption from the stomach is somewhat less than that from the small intestine. In both *in vitro* and *in vivo* studies, it has been demonstrated that over 80 percent of soluble fluorides may be absorbed in 90 minutes.

Once absorbed into the body fluids, two major mechanisms serve to reduce the fluoride concentration in the circulating body fluids:

1. Deposition in the skeleton
2. Excretion in the urine.

Routes of Intake

These are by way of the lungs (inspired air), fluids and solids.

Air

Unusual concentrations of fluoride in air are found near factories producing steel or aluminum, where fluoride is used in the process, or where fluoride-containing minerals like cryolite (Na_3AlF_6) are being mined and processed. The effluent from the stacks of steel or aluminum factories usually contain HF as a source of fluoride, but adequate scrubbers have been installed so that little appears in the air. In the case of mines producing and processing fluoride compounds like cryolite, respirators or masks may be worn to reduce exposure to dust containing fluorides. Normally, air would contain about $0.1\mu g$ fluoride per cu m, whereas concentrations as high as 3mg/cu m have been inspired by workers in an aluminum factory. The absorption of fluoride can be estimated from bone and urinary fluoride data. That is, where fluoride absorption increases due to greater intakes, more would be found in the urine. In addition, bones obtained at autopsy would show increased levels of fluoride. In a cryolite factory, Roholm has shown increased bone density on x-ray in highly exposed individuals to a degree such that the condition was diagnosed as osteosclerosis.

Fluoride containing gases or dust particles when inhaled are absorbed rather quickly, as seen by the rapid increase in urinary fluoride. This is particularly true when HF is inhaled. Adults experimentally breathing air containing about 3 ppm HF will excrete about 15 mg fluoride per day, when the normal urinary output would be about 0.1 to 0.2 mg fluoride in a nonfluoride area or 1.0 to 1.5 mg fluoride in individuals drinking water containing 1 ppm fluoride.

Water

Soluble, inorganic fluorides are rapidly absorbed, about 80 percent of the intake being found in the urine in rather carefully determined balance experiments. Some compounds which have been used for the fluoridation of municipal water supplies are NaF, Na_2SiF_6, $(NH_4)_2SiF_6$, and HF. CaF_2 in dilute solution is also quite readily absorbed. Some fluoride may exist in complexed form, which, although even more rapidly absorbed than ionic fluoride, is not metabolized and is inert physiologically. Examples of these are KPF_6 and KBF_4. A study has shown that when $200\mu g$ of NaF, Na_2SiF_6, Na_2PO_3F was introduced into the stomach of starved adult rats, about 50 percent remained in the gastrointestinal tract after 30 minutes. Only about 25 percent of KPF_6 or KBF_4, however, remained after the same length of time.

Tea

Tea leaves, and incidentally the leaves of the camellia plant (tea family), contain very high concentrations of fluoride, 90 percent of which is extracted by boiling water and hence is rapidly absorbed. Tea may contain well over 100 ppm fluoride. It is estimated that about ten cups of tea per day would be equivalent to drinking water containing 1 ppm fluoride.

Milk

Fluoride is absorbed somewhat more slowly from milk than from water, but over a four-hour period about the same total amount is absorbed.

Solids

There is some evidence to indicate that absorption from gastrointestinal tract of fluoride in food or diet is somewhat slower than absorption of sodium fluoride in water. The fluoride of bone meal is one-third to one-half as available for absorption as is a comparable amount of fluoride as NaF.

DEPOSITION

The following values refer to fluoride concentrations in a number of mineralized structures, soft tissues and body fluids. Data on the mineralized structures are expressed on a dry or dry, fat-free basis where water-borne fluoride is about 0.3 ppm.

1. Bones—500 ppm (see Fig. 9). It is estimated that fetal bones at term contain about 20 ppm fluoride.

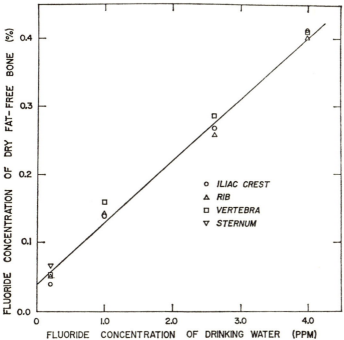

Figure 9. Relation of fluoride concentration of human bone to fluoride concentration of drinking water.

2. Cartilage—30 ppm
3. Teeth
   a. Enamel—100 ppm
   b. Dentin—300 ppm
   c. Cementum—1000 ppm
   d. Pulp—680 ppm
   e. Plaque—67 ppm
   f. Calculus
      1. Dental
         a. Supragingival—390 ppm
         b. Subgingival—240 ppm
      2. Urinary—3100 ppm
      3. Biliary—20 ppm

The concentration of fluoride decreases from the enamel surface to the dentino-enamel junction. Concentration of fluoride then increases from the dentino-enamel junction to the pulp.

It is estimated that whole fetal teeth taken at term contain about 15 ppm fluoride.

4. Soft tissues—About 1 ppm or less is found in most tissues on a fresh weight basis except for the aorta, which may contain ten times as much fluoride.

The fluoride content of the placenta tends to increase with age, due to the appearance of calcific areas near term.

5. Body fluids

  a. Blood—0.1 ppm. There is evidence from at least two independent laboratories that about 80 to 90 percent of the fluoride is "bound" and the remainder is ionic. The concentration of total fluoride in blood does not appear to change until the concentration of fluoride in the drinking water exceeds 2.5 ppm fluoride. Fetal and maternal blood contain about 0.1 to 0.2 ppm fluoride.

  b. Saliva—0.1 ppm

  c. Bile—0.1 ppm

  d. Cerebrospinal Fluid—0.1 ppm

  e. Milk—0.1 ppm

Factors Affecting Deposition

Age

1. Bones—Human rib shows an increase with age, reaching a plateau at 50 to 60 years (see Fig. 10).

2. Teeth

  a. Enamel—Concentration of fluoride increases up to 30 to 40 years and levels off (see Fig. 11).

  b. Dentin—Concentration of fluoride increases up to 50 to 60 years and then levels off (see Fig. 12).

Thus, for bones and teeth, self-limiting factors appear to operate, so that an age is reached subsequent to which little if any additional fluoride is incorporated in the bones and teeth.

Additional data are available in the rat, but not in the human, that as bones and teeth age without prior exposure

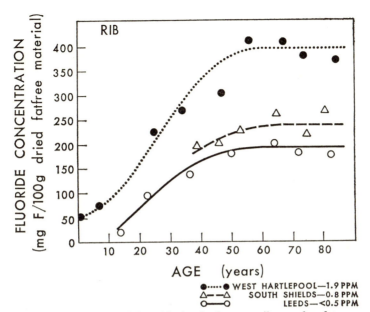

Figure 10. Concentration of fluoride in the human rib as related to age and fluoride exposure in the drinking water. ● · · · · ● West Hartlepool, 1.9 ppm fluoride △ – – △ South Shields, 0.8 ppm fluoride 0—0 Leeds, <0.5 ppm fluoride. (Courtesy Drs. Jackson and Weidmann [1958] *J. Pathol. Bact.*)

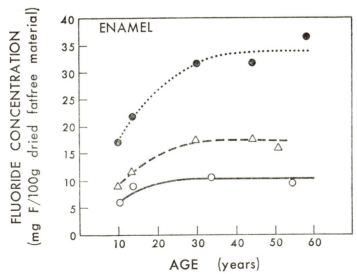

Figure 11. The relationship between age and fluoride content of human premolar enamel at various levels of fluoride exposure in the drinking water. ● · · · · ● West Hartlepool, 1.9 ppm fluoride △ – – △ South Shields, 0.8 ppm fluoride 0—0 Leeds, <0.5 ppm fluoride. (Courtesy Drs. Jackson and Weidmann [1959] *Br. Dent. J.*)

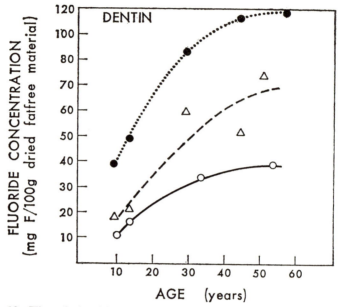

Figure 12. The relationship between age and fluoride content of human premolar dentin at various levels of exposure of fluoride in the drinking water. ●·····● West Hartlepool, 1.9 ppm fluoride △--△ South Shields, 0.8 ppm fluoride 0—0 Leeds, <0.5 ppm fluoride. (Courtesy Drs. Jackson and Weidmann [1959] *Br. Dent. J.*)

to fluoride, they lose their capacity to incorporate fluoride when it is administered.

Diet

Low-calcium diets enhance fluoride deposition and high calcium or aluminum intakes enhance excretion of fluoride in the feces, thus decreasing fluoride absorption.

Vitamin C administration is said to increase fluoride deposition, but the data are equivocal.

Increased food intake is said to increase fluoride deposition, but the data are meager in the human.

High protein intakes increase the excretion of urine and appear to produce some "washing out" effect so that the fluoride content of bone is less.

Vascularity and Turnover Rate

Where bone is turning over rapidly, as in the epiphyses, and where there is an increased blood supply, the concentration of fluoride appears to increase.

Alteration in Physiological Processes

1. Semi-starvation—A smaller bone is produced having a higher concentration of fluoride than the bones of *ad libitum* fed rats, but the total amount deposited is the same.

2. Rickets—In experimental rickets, the bone is much smaller, the concentration of fluoride is markedly elevated, but the total amount of fluoride in the rachitic bone is still less than that deposited in normal bone.

3. Diabetes—Increased water intake characteristic of untreated diabetes decreases renal tubular resorption so that fluoride would be cleared at a faster rate.

4. Kidney Disease—If the disease is advanced to a degree where there is some shutdown in urinary excretion rate, an increase in bone fluoride should result. This would probably not be greater than twofold. It has been shown that no untoward histological or chemical changes are seen in bone even when the fluoride concentration increases some eightfold in the bone.

Effect of Fluoride on Bone and Tooth Chemistry

Even with some eightfold increase in bone fluoride in humans, no changes are seen in the major components, calcium and phosphorus. Magnesium seems to increase about 10 percent and carbonate decreases a like amount. The most striking change in human bone, as also observed in the rat, the mouse, the cow and the chicken, is a decrease in citrate concentration of about 30 percent. The concentration of fluoride in the bones of individuals from a low fluoride area (<1.0 ppm) was 0.05 percent, and in the bones of individuals from a high fluoride area (4.0 ppm) was 0.40 percent.

Data on the effect of fluoride on the dental tissues is

equivocal. One laboratory found a trend toward an inverse relationship between fluoride in enamel and citrate and carbonate. The second laboratory found no relation between the fluoride concentration in enamel and its carbonate, citrate or magnesium content. No change between fluoride in enamel and carbonate was reported by a third laboratory.

MOBILIZATION

Mobilization is the release of previously deposited fluoride from calcified tissues.

Fluoride is rapidly deposited in bone as the chief reservoir. Indeed, about 95 percent of the fluoride in the body is in bone. Radioisotope work with ^{18}F is limited in view of its short half-life of about 109 minutes. There are other radioisotopes of fluoride, but they are even more short-lived.

Data in the rat indicate quite clearly that at physiological levels of fluoride intake, some 85 to 90 percent of the deposited fluoride is retained by the bones after discontinuance of administration of this ion in either the growing or the adult rat.

No direct data are available in the human, although information may be obtained in this regard from urinary studies already reported. For some 50 years or more, Bartlett, Texas, had 8 ppm fluoride in the drinking water. The urinary concentration of fluoride approached 8 ppm. When the water supply was defluoridated to 1 ppm, urine samples were collected at intervals for some 113 weeks. It would have been expected that the urinary concentration would stabilize at about 1 ppm fluoride; however, it reached an apparent steady state at about 2 ppm, indicating that the bones may have been "leaking" small amounts of fluoride. Balance data in the human indicate that over 90 percent of the fluoride deposited in the bone is retained following ingestion of various amounts of fluoride. That is, the intake of fluoride was measured, then discontinued. Fluoride excretion in the urine and feces was measured during administration of fluoride and at periods after its discontinuance.

The concentration of fluoride in the urine and feces after administration of fluoride was stopped was very low, indicating a very high retention of fluoride and hence a very low mobilization.

EXCRETION

The three main avenues for the elimination of fluoride from the body are the urine, feces and perspiration. Saliva may serve as another mode of excretion, but it is swallowed and thus recycled. The concentration of fluoride is about 0.1 to 0.2 ppm and is little affected by increased concentrations of fluoride in the drinking water. Fluoride is also found in milk in small concentrations approaching 0.1 ppm, as already mentioned, and is little affected by intake.

Urine and Feces

Urine serves as an excellent indicator of fluoride intake in the adult. The concentration of fluoride in adult urine reflects the concentration of fluoride in the water drunk within 24 to 28 hours. When an adult moves from one community to another where the concentration of fluoride varies and spot samples of urine are collected, the concentration of fluoride in the urine approaches that in his drinking water within 24 to 28 hours. In children five to 14 years of age, drinking water containing 1 ppm fluoride, the urinary concentration of fluoride did not reach 1 ppm for two to three years after the start of fluoridation. Adults reached 1 ppm fluoride within one to two weeks. It should be remembered that these types of experiments involve the analysis of isolated samples of urine. When the intake of fluoride is measured and the amounts excreted in 24-hour samples of urine and feces are recorded, then accurate data regarding the absorption can be obtained as described earlier. In young adults consuming 4 to 5 mg fluoride per day, it is estimated that about 70 percent was excreted in the urine, about 15 percent in the feces, and about 15 percent in the perspiration, so that little storage occurred.

Hence, the balances, or intake minus output, was essentially zero.

Other workers have indicated that a positive balance for fluoride may occur in that the difference between intake of fluoride and output is a positive value.

In adults averaging about 44 years of age receiving 13.0 mg fluoride per day, 7.5 mg were found in the urine and 0.9 mg in the stool, thus giving a net balance of 5.6 mg, indicating appreciable storage. Excretion in the perspiration was disregarded, and this is valid in temperate climates, since it takes elevated temperatures to produce an appreciable elimination in the sweat. When the intake of fluoride was 4.4 mg/day, the excretion in the urine and feces was 2.2 and 0.3 mg fluoride respectively with a balance then of 1.9 mg fluoride.

In another study, the fluoride intake from water containing 1 ppm fluoride was measured and the amount excreted at various intervals thereafter was also measured. A challenge dose of 5 mg fluoride in the drinking water was then given and again samples of urine were taken at the same times as during the control periods (see Fig. 13). It may be seen that the kidney responds very rapidly to the increased fluoride challenge. Indeed, during the first three hours, 20 percent of the challenge dose is excreted in the urine, and in an additional nine hours the rate of excretion has returned to the control or the "pre-challenge" state.

Perspiration

Although 24-hour studies have not been done and would indeed be difficult, concentrations of about 0.3 to 0.4 ppm fluoride is expected in the perspiration under normal conditions. When the temperature goes up to 85° F, about 15 percent of the excreted fluoride may be found in the perspiration and at more elevated temperatures, as much as 50 percent of the excreted fluoride may be in the sweat. In these cases, the proportion of fluoride in the urine is decreased.

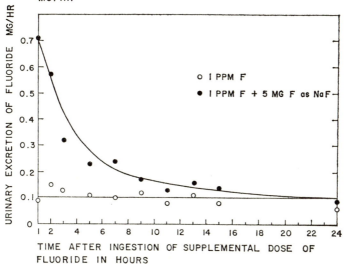

Figure 13. Urinary excretion of fluoride in eight normal individuals drinking water containing 1 ppm fluoride and receiving a supplement of 5 mg fluoride as NaF mg per hr.

MEDICAL USE OF FLUORIDE

In Bone Resorptive Diseases in the Human

Increased trabeculation of the long bones has been observed in 10 to 15 percent of an adult population drinking water containing 8 ppm fluoride for about 50 years or more. Denser bone was also seen in individuals exposed to high levels of fluoride compounds inhaled in dust. These studies and others prompted a number of clinical studies in the human in such resorptive bone diseases as osteoporosis, Paget's disease, and multiple myeloma. In many of these cases the patients are in negative calcium balance, that is, balance studies on calcium intake and excretion indicate more is excreted than is consumed. This extra calcium is coming from bone. Some 35 to 40 human studies have indicated that when as much as 1 mg fluoride per day per kg is given by mouth in divided doses, the retention of ingested calcium improves and some individuals go into positive calcium balance. In addition, increased bone density is observed on x-ray in a number of patients. It is felt that fluoride decreases the turnover of calcium as shown by isotope studies. Data indicate that there is also an improvement in the crystallinity of bone apatite, rendering it more stable.

It should be emphasized that not all the studies uniformly agree that fluoride is effective in altering calcium balance and in increasing bone density. It is questionable at this point whether the bone disease itself is clinically improved as far as the patient is concerned. No claim for the cure of the bone diseases is implied in any of the papers. It is significant that in many cases of bone resorptive diseases, bone pain is alleviated following fluoride intake.

Fish Protein Concentrate (FPC)

This material is prepared from whole fish which is extracted with isopropyl alcohol to give an almost white and almost odorless product which has almost no "fish" taste. It is very high in protein value, and preparations from a number of fishes contain over 200 ppm fluoride. The Food and Drug Administration has felt that this amount of fluoride might produce objectionable dental fluorosis. It is quite agreed that FPC would provide a good supplement for enhancing protein consumption in children on inadequate levels of protein intake.

Recent investigations in animals have shown that the fluoride of FPC as anticipated is less biologically available since it is present in the bones of the fish in a partially sequestered form as fluorapatite. A report on the incorporation of fluoride into mineralized tissues has shown that only about one-third to one-half of the fluoride in FPC is available when compared with fluoride of sodium fluoride.

To date, no human studies have been published on the effect of FPC on dental fluorosis or caries.

Organically Bound Fluorine

Fluorine may be present in such organic compounds as insecticides, refrigerant gases, steroids and anesthetics. In the past, the toxicity of these compounds has been related to the compound itself, rather than to release of fluoride. Recent studies have shown that fluoride appears in high concentration in blood and urine of individuals receiving methoxyflurane, a rather widely used anesthetic. Little is known of the capacity of various tissues, either *in vitro* or *in vivo* to enzymatically cleave fluorine in organically bound components.

These types of studies are important clinically but essentially are outside the scope of metabolism of fluoride as related to water fluoridation.

QUESTIONS FOR DISCUSSION

1. How would you distinguish between active and passive transport, that is, simple diffusion from active transport?

2. Describe an *in vivo* experiment to compare the rate of absorption of fluoride from sodium fluoride and CF_3COONa.

3. How can you reconcile the observations that fluoride in bone increases markedly as the fluoride concentration in the drinking water increases up to 2.5 ppm fluoride, while the concentration of total fluoride in the blood does not appear to change?

4. How can you account for the very low concentration of fluoride in most soft tissues (aorta excluded) and in body fluids? Speculate on the high concentrations usually found in the aorta.

5. Most but not all of the fluoride deposited in bone is retained after the administration of fluoride is stopped. What speculations can be made about the state of fluoride in bone? Would you hazard a guess on the mobilization of fluoride from teeth?

6. Calculate the concentration of fluoride in the skeleton, given the following data and assumptions:

    a. The individual weighs 70 kg

    b. The water contains 1 ppm fluoride

    c. 1000 ml water per day are consumed for 70 years

    d. 50 percent of the intake of fluoride is deposited in the skeleton

    e. 5 percent of the body weight is skeleton

    f. Ingestion of fluoride from nonliquid sources is negligible.

FURTHER READING

Brudevold, F.: 1962. Chemical composition of the teeth in relation to caries. In R.F. Sogannaes (Ed.): *Chemistry and Prevention of Dental Caries.* Springfield, Thomas, p. 32.

Hodge, H.C. and Smith, F.A.: 1965. In J.H. Simons (Ed.): *Fluorine Chemistry.* New York, Academic Press, vol. 4.

Hodge, H.C. and Smith, F.A.: 1968. Fluorides and man. *Annu. Rev. Pharmacol., 8:*395–408.

Jackson, D. and Weidmann, S.M.: 1958. The relationship of human bone as related to age and water supply of different regions. *J. Pathol. Bacteriol. 76:*451–459.

Jackson, D. and Weidmann, S.M.: 1959. The relationship between age and fluorine content of human dentine and enamel: a regional survey. *Br. Dent. J., 107:*303–306.

Largent, E.J.: 1961. *Fluorosis.* Columbus, Ohio State Univ. Press.

McClure, F.J.: 1962. *Fluoride Drinking Waters.* Public Health Service Publication Number 825.

Roholm, K.: 1937. *Fluorine Intoxication.* London, H.K. Lewis.

Smith, F.A. (Ed.): 1966. *Pharmacology of Fluorides.* New York, Springer-Verlag, vol. 20, part 1.

World Health Organization: 1970. *Fluorides and Human Health.* Monograph Number 59. Geneva, Switzerland.

Zipkin, I.: 1966. The metabolism and safety of fluorides. In A.E. Nizel (Ed.): *The Science of Nutrition and Its Application in Clinical Dentistry.* pp. 111–124.

Zipkin, I. and Babeaux, W.L.: 1965. Maternal transfer of fluoride. *J. Oral Therap. Pharmacol., 1*:652–665.

Chapter 7

FLUORIDE TOXICOLOGY

HAROLD C. HODGE

SAFETY OF WATER FLUORIDATION

O NLY THE BIOLOGICAL aspects of the safety of water fluoridation will be considered. Engineering, ethical, or legal questions have been discussed in previous chapters.

Many effects have been attributed to fluoridated drinking water, e.g. the list taken from Spira's writings which includes effects supposedly mediated through the central nervous system (depression; melancholy; changes in hair, nails, teeth and skin; blisters and cracks in the oral mucosa) and via the endocrines (adrenals—skin pigmentation, lowered blood pressure, lassitude; sex glands—feminized male) as well as effects supposedly mediated through the peripheral nervous system (neuralgia, cramps, pins and needles, numbness).

Several fluoride properties have been studied carefully enough to permit quantitative statements of dose versus response. These properties are reviewed briefly under the heading "Highlights of Fluoride Toxicology," and in the tabulation (Table XII) which follows.

TABLE XII

RESPONSES TO FLUORIDE

Concentration or Dose of Fluoride	Medium	Time	Effect
1 ppb (0.001 ppm)	Air	Lifetime	Limit for susceptible plants
1 ppm	Water	Lifetime	Dental caries reduction
2 ppm or more	Water	During tooth formation	Dental fluorosis
5 ppm	Water or air	Yrs	No osteosclerosis
8 ppm	Water	Yrs	10% osteosclerosis
20–80 mg/day or more	Water or air	Yrs	Crippling fluorosis
50 ppm	Food or water	Yrs	Thyroid changes
100 ppm	Food or water	Mos	Growth retardation
>125 ppm	Food or water	Mos	Kidney changes
2.5–5.0 gm	Acute dose	2–4 Hrs	Death

106

HIGHLIGHTS OF FLUORIDE TOXICOLOGY

The continued and increasing use of fluorides makes timely a brief resumé of some of the highlights of fluoride toxicology.

Fluoride, biologically, is a ubiquitous bone seeker with a variety of physiologic and toxic effects, some of which constitute substantial hazards if neglected, but also with properties which permit a ready control of the hazards and an assurance of safety. Six properties have been so well studied that they may serve as landmarks of fluoride toxicology; these will be discussed in some detail.

Acute Poisoning

The certainly lethal dose for the standard 70 kg adult man is estimated to be 2,500 to 5,000 mg fluoride. Because sodium fluoride is roughly half fluoride, the lethal dose is 5 to 10 gm of sodium fluoride or 1 to 2 teaspoonfuls (Hodge and Smith, 1965). The course of acute poisoning is rapid. Taken orally, death often occurs in two to four hours; many patients who live longer than four hours recover. The reasons for the rapidity are not hard to find: in high concentrations fluoride is a powerful metabolic inhibitor. Rapid absorption and rapid distribution throughout the body of a lethal or near lethal dose quickly permit dangerously high concentrations of fluoride ion to develop. Patients surviving for four or more hours have an improved prognosis because fluoride is rapidly deposited in the skeleton and rapidly excreted in the urine, thereby decreasing blood and tissue concentrations below fatal levels.

The remarkable ability of the body to dispose of fluoride accounts for the fact that large (but not lethal) doses of fluoride may be tolerated without severe toxic symptoms. For example, in unsuccessful chemotherapeutic trials some years ago, one patient suffering from leukemia received as much as 23 mg fluoride per kg intravenously daily for nine days without apparent toxic effects. Each such dose must have exceeded a quarter of the acute lethal dose given by mouth. Toxic doses of fluorides taken orally have a salty or soapy taste; nausea, vomiting, diarrhea, cramping develop promptly; with large enough doses, collapse, coma and death ensue. Death is usually attributed to a blockage of necessary enzyme or transport systems; which such system(s) are responsible for death cannot be said. Calcium-binding by overwhelming doses of fluoride probably accounts for the unclotted state of the blood reported in some autopsy examinations.

Kidney

When experimental animals are maintained for periods of months on diets or on drinking water containing over 100 ppm fluoride, various changes in kidney structure and function can be demonstrated. Tubular cells die and regenerate, interstitial fibrosis develops, and in some animals a remarkable dilatation of certain tubules begins in the loop of Henle, later involving the distal convoluted tubule (Pindborg, 1956). Such dilated tubules have not been reported in man; in fact, the only kidney effects ascribed to prolonged human exposures to fluorides are those in certain hospitalized patients in India or China with diagnoses of skeletal fluorosis who exhibited reduced kidney function (e.g. urea clearance) (Siddiqui, 1955). These patients were poverty-stricken laborers from small villages, chronically malnourished, and afflicted with various intercurrent diseases. The causative role of fluoride in their kidney impairment has by no means been established. In certain patients suffering from advanced kidney disease or in animals with specifically injured kidneys (such as occurs in uranium poisoning), the ability to excrete fluoride in the urine is not seriously impaired until the kidneys fail. In terminal uremia, fluoride is excreted more slowly than usual, blood fluoride levels increase, and as a result, the concentrations of fluoride in the skeleton increase markedly.

Thyroid

Many studies have been made of the effects of fluoride on the thyroid, perhaps partly because fluoride's being a halogen raised the question whether fluoride, like iodine, might be taken up preferentially and stored by the thyroid. It is not. Perhaps interest in the thyroid has continued because textbooks have quoted an observation made years ago of a struma or goiter in a dog repeatedly given very large doses of fluoride. Large amounts of fluoride do alter the thyroid. More than 50 ppm fluoride in the ration or drinking water administered over periods of days to years have been responsible for structural or functional changes in the thyroid in a number of species of animals. When the diets contained less than 50 ppm of fluoride, few thyroid alterations were found. The question whether fluoride is associated with human goiter can be answered simply. If the drinking water contains practically none or up to 3 ppm of fluoride in areas where iodine is deficient, goiters develop regardless of the fluoride content of the water. On the other hand, when iodine is given in such areas, for example as iodized salt, whether the drinking water contains only a trace or up to several parts per million of fluoride, the prophylactic effect of iodine is exerted. There is no direct relation of fluoride to goiter in such exposures.

Growth

The dairy cow, the most sensitive species, given a ration containing 40 ppm of fluoride for four or five years will lose weight and become unthrifty. Other species studied sustain growth impairment only with higher levels of dietary fluoride. If a single report by Japanese investigators is discounted, no adverse effects on human growth are known.

In this study, the heights and weights of children living in two small settlements in a mountainous area of Japan were compared. For one group living up the mountainside, the water supply obtained from shallow wells presumably contained excess fluoride because teeth were mottled. The children in this settlement were somewhat shorter and weighed somewhat less at a given age than the children living below in the valley whose teeth were not mottled and where presumably the fluoride intake was lower. The lack of specific information on the fluoride intake, on fluoride excretion, on the nutritional status, on the hereditary background, and of other pertinent information about these two groups prevents acceptance of the investigator's conclusion that fluoride was responsible for the growth difference.

On the other hand, reliable evidence of the normal growth of children in a fluoridated community has been gathered. Possible growth effects of fluoride consumed at 1 ppm in the drinking water were sought during a period of ten years in the two cities of Newburgh and Kingston, New York. The water supply of Newburgh was fluoridated, one of the earliest in the country; Kingston with about 0.05 ppm in the community drinking water was maintained as a control city. Thorough examinations of hundreds of children annually showed beyond doubt that growth, as revealed by height, weight, bone age estimated from wrist and knee radiographs, and by other indices, was exactly comparable in the Newburgh and in the Kingston children (Schlesinger *et al.*, 1956). A few more cortical defects were found in the radiographs of the bones of the Newburgh children; in the opinion of the radiologist, Dr. Caffey, the difference was within the limits of normal variation.

The question of adverse effects on reproduction has been examined. Large doses of fluoride interfere with fertility and normal reproductive performance. Pregnant animals of several species have been fed fluoride without teratogenic effects. Relatively large doses of fluorides to female rats during gestation caused changes in the jaw bone and in the teeth of neonatal rats.

Chronic Fluorosis

Crippling fluorosis was first described as an industrial disease. Certain workmen handling powdered cryolite in a

Danish factory developed a "poker back," characterized by a fixation of the spine. X-ray examination showed (1) that the broad ligaments had calcified; (2) that the skeleton exhibited generalized hypermineralization with moth-eaten areas of hypomineralization; and (3) that exostoses projected both from flat and from long bones (Roholm, 1937). Crippling fluorosis developed when men inhaled as dust 20 to 80 or perhaps more mg fluoride per day for protracted periods, perhaps ten to 20 years (Möller and Gudjonsson, 1932). This readily preventable illness should never recur. When fluoride exposures are unavoidable, urine analyses offer a reliable quantitative index of the exposures. The lengthy latent period permits the degree of exposure to be identified and controlled by appropriate safety measures. Radiographic examination will reveal asymptomatic osteosclerosis long before joint function is impaired. Skeletal fluoride is mobilized and slowly removed from the body when exposure is reduced.

Interest has recently heightened in the possibility of using fluorides to induce new bone formation, in treating osteoporosis, or more importantly as a prophylactic agent against it (Hodge and Smith, 1968). Large doses of fluoride, 30 to 100 mg fluoride per day, produced in some patients with osteoporosis or other bone lesions a positive calcium balance, a reduction in skeletal calcium 47 retention, and ultimately the formation of new bone which although abnormal may at least have a splinting effect. A major health benefit to the elderly would accrue if the fluoride in community drinking water (especially at elevated concentrations) lessened the incidence of spontaneously occurring osteoporosis.

Some encouraging evidence to this effect was recently gathered in North Dakota by comparing the incidence in the northwestern part of the state where certain community drinking water supplies contain 3 to 6 ppm fluoride with that in the southeastern part where drinking water supplies contain 0.1 to 0.3 ppm fluoride (Bernstein *et al.*, 1966). A radiographic survey of about 1,000 individuals in these two areas showed a lessened incidence of osteoporosis with age in women living in the high fluoride area. No such contrast was noted among the men. Unexpectedly, calcification of the aorta was markedly reduced both in men and women in the high fluoride areas.

Preliminary studies of the osteosclerotic changes have by no means clarified the mechanism of this effect. Recent attempts to understand the mechanism have produced several remarkable findings.

1. The rapidity of calcium 47 deposition in the skeleton of osteoporotic subjects was reduced after prolonged fluoride treatment, i.e. less bone participated in the rapid exchange (Neer *et al.*, 1966). Remineralization, or new bone formation, which reduced the amount of bone "available" to the circulation would plausibly account for such a difference.

2. A narrowing of the x-ray diffraction peaks of the bones of fluoride-treated men or animals is interpreted as an increase in the average crystal size of the apatite mineral (Bernstein and Cohen, 1967). Larger crystals possess smaller surface to weight ratios and have, therefore, less exchangeable calcium. Furthermore, the dissolution rates of larger crystals are less than of smaller ones, an effect which together with the considerably lower solubility attributed to the fluorapatite lattice would contribute greater "stability" to bone. The role of these factors in the reduced osteoporosis of elderly women (see above) has not been evaluated nor has it in the new bone formation either in chronic fluorosis or in fluoride-treated osteoporotic patients.

3. Paradoxically, prolonged treatment with large doses of fluoride *reduces* the incorporation of proline into bone collagen (Proffit and Ackerman, 1964). Carbon 14-hydroxyproline tends to accumulate in the cell rather than in collagen. Such an interference with osteocytic metabolism would be expected to accompany a *reduction* in new bone formation. Perhaps this effect accounts for the fact that in patients suffering from crippling fluorosis certain local

areas of bone may become hypomineralized; in these areas, described as moth eaten, bone formation is notably impaired.

4. Several observations direct attention to an intriguing possibility that the parathormone is somehow involved in the osteosclerotic response to repeated large doses of fluoride. The parathyroid gland enlarges and becomes hyperplastic in sheep and in rabbits receiving 200 ppm fluoride in their rations (Faccini, 1967). The rat seems not to be responsive; at any rate, rat bone whether it contains extra fluoride or not serves successfully as a source of calcium when parathormone is put into the tissue culture. According to a complicated hypothesis, the parathyroid-mediated osteosclerosis involves two sequences. First, *parathyroid stimulation*. Fluoride deposited in bone renders the bone calcium somewhat less available, thereby lowering slightly the concentration of blood calcium which stimulates parathormone secretion, increasing the activity of the bone cells and reestablishing the normal blood calcium. Second, *increased collagen formation*. Recent preliminary evidence indicates that a secondary effect of parathyroid stimulation occurring later than the well-established mobilization of bone mineral may, under certain circumstances, be a speeded-up collagen formation. In an animal chronically exposed to excessive amounts of fluoride, new bone formation might follow.

The brightest aspect of these sophisticated attempts to understand how toxic doses of fluoride alter the structure and function of bone may well be not these and other findings but the enthusiasm of the attack.

FURTHER READING

Bernstein, D.S. and Cohen, P.: 1967. Use of sodium fluoride in the treatment of osteoporosis. *J. Clin. Endocrinol. Metab.*, 27:197–210.

Bernstein, D.S., Sadowsky, N., Hegsted, D.M., Guri, C.D. and Stare, F.J.: 1966. Prevalence of osteoporosis in high- and low-fluoride areas in North Dakota. *J.A.M.A.*, 198:499–504.

Faccini, J.M.: 1967. Inhibition of bone resorption in the rabbit by fluoride. *Nature*, 214:1269–1271.

Hodge, H.C. and Smith, F.A.: 1965. In J.H. Simons (Ed.) : *Fluorine Chemistry.* New York, Academic Press, vol. 4.

Hodge, H.C. and Smith, F.A.: 1968. Fluorides and man. *Annu. Rev. Pharmacol., 8:*395–408.

Möller, P.F. and Gudjonsson, S.V.: 1932. Massive fluorosis of bones and ligaments. *Acta Radiol., 13:*269–294.

Neer, R.M., Zipkin, I., Carbone, P.P. and Rosenberg, L.E.: 1966. Effect of sodium fluoride therapy on calcium metabolism in multiple myeloma. *J. Clin. Endocrinol. Metab., 26:*1059–1068.

Pindborg, J.J.: 1965. The effect of 0.05% dietary sodium fluoride on the rat kidney. *Acta Pharmacol. Toxicol., 13:*36–45.

Proffit, W.R. and Ackerman, J.L.: 1964. Fluoride: Its effect on two parameters of bone growth in organ culture. *Science, 145:*932–934.

Roholm, K.: 1937. *Fluorine Intoxication.* London, H.K. Lewis.

Schlesinger, E.R., Overton, D. E., Chase, H.C. and Cantwell, K.T.: 1956. Newburgh-Kingston caries-fluorine study, XIII. Pediatric findings after ten years. *J. Am. Dent. Assoc., 52:*296–306.

Siddiqui, A.H.: 1955. Fluorosis in Nalgonda district, Hyderabad-Deccan. *Br. Med. J., 2:*1408–1413.

Chapter 8

EVALUATION OF SOME OBJECTIONS TO WATER FLUORIDATION

H.C. HODGE

Dr. KENNETH R. ELWELL with Dr. Kenneth A. Easlick has prepared an 82-page booklet entitled *Classification and Appraisal of Objections to Fluoridation* (University of Michigan, School of Public Health, 1960). Eight categories cover 137 specific objections; pertinent bibliographic reference lists accompany each category.

The British Dental Association in February 1963, published a somewhat similar compilation under the title: *Fluoridation of Water Supplies, Questions and Answers* (13 Hill St., Berkeley Square, London, Wl). Eighteen dental questions, 40 medical questions and 13 miscellaneous questions are answered.

A few of these questions and objections will be discussed in some detail herewith.

CANCER

Alfred Taylor has published the results of two experiments on tumor-bearing mice from which he concluded that fluoride (1) decreased life span, or (2) accelerated tumor growth.

The first studies (1954) examined the life spans of groups of female mice of two strains, a high mammary cancer strain, C₃H, and a low cancer strain, dba. In the first group of experiments the mice were maintained on a Purina chow diet and received distilled water containing 0 to 10 ppm fluoride. It was discovered that the Purina diet contained 20 to 38 ppm fluoride. Therefore in the second group of experiments the mice were fed a mixed grain diet containing "negligible" fluoride. The data from his second experiments are shown in Table XIII. He concluded that fluoride in the drinking water reduced the life span by 9 percent and that this was a general effect irrespective of the fluoride in the solid diet, of the strain, or the age of the animal. There was no significant difference between the group drinking 1 and 10 ppm fluoride.

Armstrong and Bittner of the University of Minnesota repeated Taylor's studies but were unable to demonstrate a reduction in life span.

In his second study (1965) Taylor followed the growth of mouse tumor tissue implanted in mice or incubated eggs. The tumor was a mammary adenocarcinoma. Fluoride was introduced in the mouse-tumor system either by addition to the tumor-saline preparation before injection, to the drink-

TABLE XIII

RELATIONSHIP BETWEEN LIFE SPAN AND SODIUM FLUORIDE IN THE DRINKING WATER OF MICE ON A PURINA DIET

	No. of Mice	Strain of Mice	Fluoride Conc. (ppm)	Avg. Life Span, Control = 100	Deaths, Period of Exp. (1%)
C	24	C₃H	0	100	71
E	24	C₃H	1	83.6	96
E	24	C₃H	10	102.7	79
C	24	dba	0	100	54
E	24	dba	1	92.7	67
E	24	dba	10	92.1	62
C	42	dba	0	100	75
E	42	dba	1	90.5	78
E	42	dba	10	91.9	86
C	12	C₃H	0	100	80
E	12	C₃H	1	93.8	92
E	12	C₃H	10	86.6	100
C	28	C₃H	0	100	72
E	29	C₃H	1	84.9	72
			Avg.	C 100	71
				E 91	81

C = control
E = experimental
(* Courtesy Dr. Taylor [1965] *Proc. Soc. Exp. Biol. Med.*)

ing water of the experimental animals immediately after inoculation with tumor tissue or by subdermal injection of sodium fluoride for four days. Taylor concluded that a significant acceleration of tumor tissue growth had occurred with comparatively low levels of sodium fluoride irrespective of the route and amount administered. Representative data from these experiments are shown in Tables XIV and XV.

Consider the fact that in the mice described in Table XIV, the most dilute inoculum contained perhaps half the fluoride concentration of normal mouse plasma, whereas the most concentrated was 250 times the plasma concentration. Both apparently stimulated tumor growth quantitatively to the same extent. No such phenomenon has previously been reported.

In Table XV, note the "stimulant" effect of 1 ppm fluoride in the drinking water of the mice and compare it quantitatively with the effects of 2 ppm, 20 ppm and 55 ppm.

TABLE XIV

NaF ADDED TO TUMOR SUSPENSIONS BEFORE IMPLANTATION AND GROWTH OF TUMOR TRANSPLANTS IN MICE

	No. Mice		Dosage mg/.2 ml Injection	Tumor Wt, Control = 100
Exp	Control	Exp		
1	9	7	.000,01	125
2	8	5	.000,01	139
3	9	8	.000,1	125
4	11	11	.000,1	106
5	9	6	.000,1	118
6	9	9	.000,1	140
7	6	5	.000,5	141
8	8	8	.000,5	163
9	7	8	.000,5	96
10	8	5	.000,5	113
11	10	9	.001	126
12	10	7	.001	103
13	10	10	.002,5	124
14	9	9	.005	144
15	9	8	.005	126
Total No. mice	132	115		

Control avg tumor wt (gm) 1.29; S.D. ± .441
Exp avg tumor wt (gm) 1.63; S.D. ± .536
Significance of difference in avg tumor wt, $P = <.001$

TABLE XV

NaF ADDED TO DRINKING WATER AND GROWTH
OF TUMOR TRANSPLANTS IN MICE

No. Mice

Exp	Control	Exp	Dosage, mg/l	Tumor Wt Control = 100
1	17	14	1	117
2	12	11	1	113
3	10	7	2	129
4	20	19	2	113
5	8	8	2	161
6	9	9	2	113
7	8	6	2	103
8	9	7	2	161
9	10	10	2	132
10	7	6	2	117
11	10	10	2	118
12	8	6	5	101
13	5	7	5	106
14	18	17	20	113
15	10	8	20	136
16	16	13	20	89
17	9	10	44	100
18	7	7	55	114
19	10	9	55	123
Total No. mice	203	184		

Control avg tumor wt (gm) .97; S.D. ± .360
Exp avg tumor wt (gm) 1.11; S.D. ± .387
Significance of differences in avg tumor wt, $P = <.013$

Berry and Trillwood of Cambridge University reported that 0.1 ppm of sodium fluoride inhibited the growth in cell culture of two lines of mammalian cells (HeLa cells of human origin and mouse fibroblasts). Taylor suggested that if greater dilutions of fluoride had been used, a stimulation might well have been discovered.

These findings have been refuted by subsequent articles which showed that no inhibition of growth in several cell cultures occurred up to about 5 ppm, whereas inhibition was detectable at 10 to 20 ppm fluoride.

Epidemiologic studies comparing the death rates from cancer have shown no significant differences, such as the 1954 report covering 32 pairs of cities in 16 states with pairings based on community water supplies containing 0.25 ppm or less versus those containing 0.7 ppm or more.

STOMATITIS

Douglas has presented a summary of clinical observations recording the incidence of stomatitis in 133 patients, all of whom used a fluoride dentifrice. His attention had been drawn to the problem by the increasing frequency of complaints of stomatitis during the preceding 15 months without a discernible causative basis. These patients ranged in age from 3 1/2 to 92 years, mostly between 20 and 60. "As many as six of a family of seven with stomatitis of fluoride origin" had been seen.

Thirty-two patients cooperated over a range of two to six courses; "each course consisted of use for three weeks of the dentifrice until normalcy had been maintained three weeks." Two patients lasted through six courses, five through five, one through four, seven through three, and 18 through two. Each time the patients began using the fluoride dentifrice, severe lesions appeared earlier and cleared with more difficulty.

"All of the 133 patients showed whitish exudate over the superficially ulcerated lesions." Seventeen had foul breath, 94 bled easily, 29 described "soreness of the teeth"—a tightness, "a peculiar feeling of the teeth not being 'set right in the socket,'" 18 described ptyalism. Bacteriologic examinations regretably were not carried out in all cases. Where done, increased staphylococcal counts were found, and in the severe cases high counts of anaerobes were found.

CONVULSIONS

The following is a case report presented by Waldbott in 1957:

"W. J., a 12-year-old boy, was admitted . . . to Harper Hospital because of tetanic convulsions involving left arm and leg only." The seizures had started over a year earlier; some days he had 25 attacks in 24 hours. He never became unconscious; there was no aura although he had some premonition such as slight headaches and stiffening of arm muscle.

Previous history was not rewarding. Physical findings were normal. Laboratory studies gave results mostly in the normal ranges. Akaline phosphatase levels ranged from 11.3 to 21 units (normal: 8 to 13). Radiographs disclosed no abnormalities.

The patient resided in Saginaw, Michigan, where many well waters contain fluoride naturally and where the community water supply had been fluoridated, but the practice was discontinued one month prior to his hospitalization. Urinary fluoride concentrations were reported: 4.4 ppm during this hospital stay, 1.0 to 1.4 ppm in four samples taken during the succeeding two years.

"Fluoride water was suspected as the precipitating cause of the convulsions." Distilled water was therefore used for cooking and drinking; foods high in fluorides (tea, seafood) were avoided.

In the following year, the patient had minor attacks at roughly monthly intervals. "The EEG showed one spike and slow wave complex in alertness, a second questionable one after hyperventilation, no evidence of an acute lesion." During the second year, an intradermal injection of 1 mg of sodium fluoride precipitated a convulsion 3 hours later, the first one in four months. A control saline injection a few days later "produced no ill effect." Eight months later, the patient suffered an episode of many seizures.

An etiologic role for fluorides was postulated on the basis of the following facts:

1. high normal blood calcium, increase in alkaline phosphatase;

2. higher urinary fluoride levels when convulsions were present;

3. minor seizure after a fluoride skin test;

4. attacks subsided while fluoride water was avoided;

5. tetaniform convulsions are a feature of acute fluoride intoxication;

6. the final episode of many seizures was assumed to have been precipitated by sudden intake of a dose of flu-

oride either from drinking fluoride-containing water, from eating fluoride-containing food, or "through inhalation from the air, or a combination of these. No information on these could be secured."

As an addendum: About a year later, the patient was given a "blindfold test." From three identical bottles, doses of 1 tablespoon were taken for five successive days. Two bottles contained distilled water, the third 1 mg of sodium fluoride in each dose. On the fifth day of dosing from the fluoride-containing bottle, a convulsive seizure occurred. Daily urinary fluoride levels, zero during the two weeks on the placebo bottles, rose to 1.5 mg/day after five days on fluoride water, and subsequently became negative again.

THE QUESTION OF FLUORIDE ALLERGY

Contact dermatitis from fluoride solutions is well known and has been encountered by incautious dentists giving topical applications. Concentrated fluoride solutions are irritants; the contact dermatitis apparently is self-limiting and disappears with removal of the irritating agent.

Reports of fluoride allergy have come principally from Waldbott, an allergist. For example, in 1956 he described the problem of a patient with early rheumatoid arthritis whose drinking water (private well) contained 0.8 ppm fluoride, and who improved when he stopped drinking this water. The disease reappeared when he took for one week, 1 tablespoonful of a fluoride solution daily (1 mg fluoride per dose) using double blind precautions. Competent immunologists have been unwilling to accept Waldbott's reports as proof of the existence of a fluoride allergy. The executive committee of the American Academy of Allergy, having reviewed clinical reports of allergy to fluoride, has adopted unanimously the following statement (Austen *et al.*, 1971) : "There is no evidence of allergy or intolerance to fluorides as used in fluoridation of community water supplies."

The recent discovery by Taves that human serum fluoride exists in two forms, exchangeable (presumably fluoride ion) and non exchangeable (traveling with and perhaps bound to albumin), gives a basis for anticipating that an allergenic substance bearing fluoride might be present in the body. At present this is only a hypothesis. The nature of the association between fluoride and albumin is unknown except that the fluoride is not acid labile. The question of what the albumin-fluoride complex is and whether it or some other fluoride complex plays a role in a sensitization to fluoride needs exploration.

ACUTE MAGNESIUM DEFICIENCY

Marier, Rose and Boulet (1963) proposed that since the magnesium content of bone increased with increasing fluoride content (with a stoichiometric relation), inadequate reserves of serum magnesium might on occasion be depleted with consequent bone injury including exostosis production. They concluded that "More research into the interrelation between magnesium and fluoride deposition appears to be desirable." The unstated inference apparently could be drawn that until this research had been completed and the hazards of magnesium deficiency shown to be negligible, water fluoridation should be postponed.

An examination of three parts of their argument in greater detail shows little solid evidence.

1. "An examination of the data of Zipkin revealed that the extent of the Mg increase was a consistent function of

TABLE XVI
VARIATION IN THE RATIO OF MAGNESIUM TO FLUORIDE IN MINERALIZED TISSUES

Tissue	Mg/Fluoride (molar ratio) *	Investigator
Human rib	0, 6, 8	Zipkin *et al.* (1960)
Human vertebra	4, 3, 7	
Rat bone	7, 12, 13	
Rat dentine	8, 2	McCann and Bullock (1957)
Rat enamel	2, 0.6	

* Each number from a separate analysis

fluoride deposition with a molar Mg/fluoride ratio of 1:8; this supports the concept of surface deposition demonstrated by Neuman." (Marier *et al., 1963*)

There exists no demonstrable constancy between the fluoride and magnesium levels of bone contrary to the statement of Marier. The range of Mg:fluoride is from 1:0.6 to 1:13 or 25-fold variation (Table XVI).

The few useful analyses show Mg:fluoride ratios of 1:3 to 1:8 for human rib and vertebra and 1:0.6 to 1:13 for rat hard tissues; these hardly are constant values.

The second step in their argument accepts a suggestion from Weidmann that MgF_2 deposits in fluorotic bone.

2. "Such a MgF_2 deposition could only involve a local excess of these ions near the bone surface, as the levels of these ions in normal serum are not high enough to exceed the solubility product of the salt." (Marier *et al.,* 1963)

With a solubility product of 2×10^{-10} for MgF_2 and extra-cellular fluid levels of about 3 mg% for magnesium (1.2×10^{-3} M) and 0.0019 mg% for fluoride ion (1×10^{-6} M) it can be calculated that the likelihood of exceeding the solubility product of MgF_2 is very small. The product of plasma (Mg) and (F)^2 is 1.2×10^{-15}. If corrections for activity rather than concentration are made, the product of plasma (Mg) and (F)^2 is 1.5×10^{-16}. Thus the formation of MgF_2 would require an increase of magnesium concentration in plasma of about 1 million times. The existence of a MgF_2 phase seems highly unlikely on solubility grounds (solubility of MgF_2 is 76 ppm at 18°).

Third, the proposed depletion of serum magnesium appears to be improbable in normal individuals.

3. "However, we believe that this uptake of Mg by bone might, in some cases, deplete inadequate reserves of serum Mg." (Marier *et al.,* 1963)

The increase in magnesium in individuals drinking water containing 4 ppm fluoride compared to those drinking water with 1 ppm of fluoride during 70 years exposure

TABLE XVII

INCREASE OF BONE MAGNESIUM WITH AGE AT TWO LEVELS OF WATER FLUORIDE CONCENTRATION

Drinking Water Fluoride (ppm)	*Bone Mg (10–80 yrs exposure)*	
	%	*gm in adult skeleton*
1	0.50	30
4	0.60	36

equals 6,000 mg (Table XVII). It can be calculated that this increase could be accomplished in ten years if 1.64 mg of magnesium were deposited daily. Dietary ingestion of magnesium normally is 270 mg per day, so that an individual would consume 6,000 mg of magnesium in the diet in 22 days. In a ten-year period he would have ingested 985,000 mg. Compare this with the fact that the total circulating level of magnesium is between 425 to 756 mg. The likelihood of causing a magnesium deficiency by ingestion of fluoride in the drinking water is so remote as to not require serious consideration.

MONGOLISM

In a propaganda sheet distributed on occasion by opponents to water fluoridation, a photograph shows a number of mongoloid children in a room, presumably a schoolroom. The propagandists aver that "a highly qualified scientist, Dr. Lionel Rapaport of the University of Wisconsin, has reported findings indicating a significant increase of mongoloid births in fluoridated communities over non-fluoridated communities." The question is then plainly put, "Can future . . . parents afford this gamble with their as yet unborn children?"

Rapaport, not a trained epidemiologist, examined birth certificates in rural areas and villages in Wisconsin, Dakota and Illinois. There is a great stream of underground water running eastward across this part of the United States bearing higher concentrations of fluoride than is found in the surface well waters. Most farmsteads have surface wells and use water low in fluoride. A good many towns have drilled deep wells to obtain additional water-supplies;

these contain as high as 2 or occasionally 3 or more ppm fluoride. Thus, a comparison can be made between two populations: (1) the farm folks drinking low fluoride water, and (2) the town folks drinking water with 1 to 3 ppm fluoride. Rapaport found (1) that the incidence of mongolism ranged from 0.13 to 0.71 per 1,000 live births in each of the three states; and (2) that there was, however, about a two-fold higher incidence of mongolism in the towns where the water contained higher fluoride concentrations (Table XVIII). To confirm or deny these findings, Russell of the U.S. Public Health Service collected data from an area in Illinois situated in the belt of fluoride-bearing deep water supplies. Ten matching counties were selected, five of them contiguous, in which shallow wells supplied the water for country dwellers. In one group of five counties, the cities mostly had water supplies containing 1.5 ppm fluoride or more. In the second group no city had a water supply with more than 0.9 ppm fluoride. Russell recorded the number of mongoloids institutionalized in the period from 1930 to 1950. The difference in the incidence of mongolism between these two groups of counties was so small that the difference could occur five out

TABLE XVIII

INCIDENCE OF MONGOLISM IN RELATION TO THE FLUORIDE CONTENT OF WATER

Location	Water Fluoride (ppm)	Incidence of Mongolism *	Investigator
Wisconsin	1.4, 2.8	0.32, 0.30	Rapaport (1956)
	0.1	.13 .18	
Dakota	>3	0.35	
	<3	0.15	
Illinois	1 –2.6	0.71	Rapaport (1959)
	0.3–0.7	0.47	
	0 –0.2	0.34	
England	0.7–4	1.42	Berry (1958)
	<0.2	1.53	
Switzerland		1.15–1.92	Various
Denmark		1.5 median	
USA			

* Mongols per 1000 births

of six times by chance. Berry in 1958 could find no difference in England in the incidence of mongolism between low fluoride and higher fluoride communities. Furthermore, Berry pointed out that in England, Switzerland, Denmark and the United States, various groups of investigators uniformly reported an incidence rate of mongolism usually of about 1.5 mongoloids per 1,000 births. Rapaport could not have recorded all the mongoloids; in other words, the design or execution of his study was at fault.

FLUORIDES VERSUS "NUTRITIONAL" PREVENTION

It has been argued that dental caries is a nutritional problem which should be solved by supplements of phosphate, or by reducing sugar intake, or by other means, not by fluorides.

Åslander hopes to see children "with lifetime teeth" like those of his own family who were given bone meal supplements from infancy. His parents (in Sweden) ate whole grilled herrings between bread, bones and all, for breakfast and had perfect teeth. In his own boyhood, herring was cooked in water and the bones carefully removed; his teeth were very poor. He was thus led to elucidate "the problem of dental caries as a deficiency disease." He argues that *partial* nutrition, for instance by supplying fluoride, cannot produce perfect teeth; therefore, water fluoridation is "an indecisive remedy."

HEMODIALYSIS WITH FLUORIDATED WATER

The safety of fluoridated water as the dialysate for patients with severe renal disease or on the artificial kidney was questioned by John Lear's article in the *Saturday Review* (March 1, 1969) following an oral presentation by Posen *et al.* before the American Society of Nephrology in November 1968. (Posen *et al.*'s paper has not yet been published.) Patients in a hospital in Ottawa, Canada, who had been dialyzed chronically with fluoridated water showed a high incidence of severe osteodystrophy not yielding to therapy with calcium and vitamin D. Their elevated serum fluorides (av. 0.36 ppm) suggested a role of fluoride in their bone disease.

Taves (personal communication) has obtained some information on a group of patients, also chronically dialyzed, in another community with a fluoridated water supply. These patients neither suffered from bone destruction nor had elevated serum fluorides.

During dialysis with fluoridated water, a patient may absorb 10 mg fluoride or more. In the absence of kidney function or in severely impaired function, most of this fluoride would be deposited in the skeleton. As expected, marked elevations in bone fluoride concentrations have been demonstrated.

Most hospitals used de-ionized water for hemodialysis.

ADVANCED KIDNEY DISEASE

Patients with kidney disease may accumulate more fluoride in their bones than do normal patients of the same age.

A few patients suffering from severe impairment of kidney function have been studied in detail, including fluoride analyses of bone samples. Osteosclerosis has been demonstrated, associated with fluoride levels of 4500 ppm or more. Two of these patients drank waters with elevated fluoride concentrations (2 to 4 ppm); one patient drank fluoridated water (1 ppm).

The patient presented by Sauerbrunn *et al.* (1965) had for years consumed large quantities of fluids (4 to 10 liters daily). A diagnosis of diabetes insipidus had been offered nearly ten years before his terminal illness. Well waters in the farming areas of Texas in which the patient had spent most of his life were naturally fluoride-bearing (2.2 to 3.5 ppm fluoride). Bone removed at autopsy contained 6100 ppm fluoride (dry weight basis). This patient's history raises a question of the hazard of fluoridated water for patients suffering from an impaired kidney function, who exhibit a slower rate of urinary fluoride excretion, and especially those with an exaggerated fluid intake, i.e. an increased daily fluoride intake.

The recently developed analytical method which discriminates between "exchangeable" fluoride (presumably fluoride ion) and "non-exchangeable" fluoride in human blood serum offers a reliable approach to the control of fluoride therapy, e.g. in osteoporosis, and also a rational index by which to detect excessive fluoride exposure and to prevent fluoride intoxication in patients, such as those in renal failure. The limited pertinent information from studies of cattle, rats and man is given in Table XIX.

Taves considers that a fasting serum fluoride of 0.1 to 0.2 ppm may predictably avoid toxic effects and yet induce beneficial mineralization of osteoporotic bone. Such a concentration range might be suggested as a tentative guide for evaluating the status of a patient with advanced renal disease and polydipsia.

TABLE XIX

RELATION OF SERUM FLUORIDE CONCENTRATIONS
TO FLUORIDE EFFECTS

Species	Serum Fluoride (ppm)	Effect or Circumstance	Investigator
Cattle	0.3	Osteoblast function altered	Carlson (1966)
	0.2	Dental fluorosis	Carlson (1966)
Rats	0.3 or more	Decreased growth, serum protein, and amino acid uptake by liver	Taves *et al.* (1970)
	1	Increased mortality	
Man	0.01 (ionic)	None; low fluoride drinking water	Taves (1968)
	0.02 (ionic)	None; 1 ppm fluoride drinking water	Taves (1968)
	0.17	Fluoride therapy (45 mg/day for 14 months) for osteoporosis	Cass *et al.* (1966)
	0.79–0.85	Fluoride therapy (100 mg/day); one patient	Armstrong *et al.* (1964)
	0.45–0.65 (1.77–single value)	Fluoride therapy (50 mg/day); one patient	Armstrong *et al.* (1964)
	0.23–0.34	Fluoride therapy (50–75 mg/day); 3 patients	Armstrong *et al.* (1964)

CAN FLUORIDE AFFECT EYESIGHT?

Large doses of sodium fluoride (40-65 mg/kg) given intravenously to rabbits induced in about one in five a marked retinal degeneration usually within 48 hours. The lesions were limited in extent sharply demarcated from the rest of the fundus. They resembled human retinitis pigmentosa.

These results were cited by Geall and Beilin (1964) as a basis for attributing to the fluoride therapy (for osteoporosis) the development of bilateral optic neuritis in a man who had received 30 mg fluoride daily for a period of six weeks. This patient, a 58-year-old man, two years earlier had developed severe thoracic backache four months after a partial gastrectomy for a chronic duodenal ulcer. Several thoracic vertebrae showed partial collapse (idiopathic osteoporosis), and his chest plate showed old pneumoconiosis and fibrotic tuberculosis contracted in the coal mines in his youth. His leg pulses were reduced; a femoropopliteal bypass graft was successful.

He was given androgen and calcium therapy for six months without improvement. A total parathyroidectomy was done and he was given androgen, calcium gluconate, calciferol and dehydrocodeine. Five months later (still no improvement) he took for six weeks 20 mg NaF, t.i.d. orally, along with his other drugs. When pain and poor vision developed, he was readmitted, NaF was stopped, and he was started on 30 mg prednisone daily. The right optic disc was edematous, the margin of the left optic disc was slightly blurred, and he had bilateral macular edema. The diagnosis—bilateral toxic neuropathy.

Waldbott had several years ago ascribed a retinopathy in one patient and incipient changes in the retina of another to the consumption of fluoridated water. No other reports are known of deleterious fluoride effects on human eyesight.

In contrast, no ocular changes were found in two other studies of 11 patients receiving fluoride therapy (30 mg fluoride daily) nor in the children of Newburgh drinking

1 ppm fluoride for ten years. Moreover, controlled studies of rabbit eyes in which doses of 20 mg NaF per kg were given daily for three to five months provided no detectable changes.

HAS FLUORIDE A ROLE IN FOG DISASTERS?

Roholm reviewed the events in the "mysterious fog disaster" of December 1930 in the densely populated Meuse Valley of Belgium. A cold, quiet fog lay in a heavy blanket under an inversion layer which held the effluents from the many factories (iron works, metal works, glass and ceramics factories, zinc works, a super phosphate plant) in the deep, narrow valley. Several thousand persons became ill with acute pulmonary symptoms, and about 60 deaths occurred in a five-day period. The dyspnea and asthma-like symptoms were attributed by an investigation commission to the irritant properties of waste gases, probably chiefly SO_2 (known to be present). Roholm pointed out (1) the irritant properties of gaseous fluorides, e.g. HF, SiF_4 and (2) the fact that 15 of the 27 factories in the valley used fluorides and presumably released gaseous fluoride compounds into the chimney smoke. He concluded that "an analysis of the details of the disaster gives circumstantial evidence that the malady was acute fluorine intoxication."

Subsequent studies discount an important role for fluoride and emphasize the possibility that zinc ammonium sulfate particles in an SO_2-containing atmosphere played a major role in "toxic fog" incidents, such as that in Donora, Pennsylvania, in 1948. Analyses of the particulate matter from a sample taken in Donora during the fog showed that of the 22 percent which was water-soluble, more than half was zinc ammonium sulfate, and one-fifth was zinc sulfate. Amdur and Corn demonstrated the remarkable ability of a combination of zinc ammonium sulfate particulate plus SO_2 to increase pulmonary resistance in experimental animals. In their opinion, if the particle size of the zinc ammonium sulfate in the Donora fog was small enough (0.3μ-0.5μ or less), this component probably contributed 'to the discomfort'.

SUMMARY

A public health measure involving the involuntary exposure of essentially the entire population of communities to a substance, such as fluoride, must reasonably be undertaken only after the most searching inquiries into its safety. Every conceivable question must be considered and evidence brought forward that no unacceptable hazard to health exists. It is impossible to prove that no one under any circumstance will ever be injured by water fluoridation. It is not only possible, it is mandatory to search vigorously and without letup for any evidence of ill effect.

Many, many questions have been raised, and many protests voiced over water fluoridation. A few scientifically valid questions for further study have been identified. Other questions based on uncontrolled or poorly controlled observations can be dismissed. Fluoride has the enormous benefit of natural occurrence in community water supplies so that demonstrations of exposures of populations for generations preceded the proposals to fluoridate at 1 ppm (in temperate climates). No injury from fluoridated water has been proven to date. Inspired surveillance must continue with unabated zeal to detect injury if it occurs.

QUESTIONS FOR DISCUSSION

1. Assuming a community drinking water supply is fluoridated at 1 ppm and (a) that an average adult drinks 1 liter of water daily, whereas (b) that an average child drinks 0.2 to 0.6 liters daily, what factors of safety can be estimated against the toxic effects described?

2. What illnesses might pose safety problems in patients drinking fluoridated water?

3. Contrast the safety problems of fluoride made available as tablets, in milk, as a dentifrice (or in other vehicles) with that of water fluoridation.

4. Suggest if you can a hypothetical basis for Taylor's cancer results: (a) in reducing life span uniformly regard-

less of the fluoride concentration in the drinking water; (b) in accelerating transplanted tumor growth regardless of the quantity of fluoride administered or the means of fluoride treatment.

5. Douglas's observations tying severe stomatitis to the use of fluoride dentifrices convinced him that a cause-effect relation existed. What additional information would you have asked Douglas to obtain to allow you to evaluate his conclusion?

6. Do you accept Walbott's diagnosis implicating fluoride as the precipitating agent in the convulsions by the 12-year-old boy? Might this case represent an idiosyncrasy to fluoride? On what system of tests would a fluoride allergy be identified?

7. Under what conditions does a magnesium deficiency develop? What are the consequences? Evaluate the hazard of precipitating a magnesium deficiency by drinking fluoridated water.

8. Do you think the interest in mongoloid children might have arisen from the often questioned relation between the thyroid and fluoride?

9. How important is nutrition in tooth health? Should efforts to increase the public health control of and eradication of dental caries center on nutrition rather than on fluorides?

10. How can fluoride induce osteosclerosis in some areas of bone and osteoporosis in others? Would you use fluoridated water in a hemodialysis unit? What threat could fluoridated drinking water pose to a patient in terminal uremia? To a patient with severe renal disease?

11. Was the fluoride responsible in your opinion for the optic effects in Geall and Beilin's patient? In Waldbott's two patients?

12. Is the presence of fluoride in a "toxic fog" enough to incriminate fluoride as the causative irritant agent?

FURTHER READING

Amdur, M.O. and Corn, M.: 1963. The irritant potency of zinc ammonium sulfate of different particle sizes. *Am. Ind. Hyg. Assoc. J., 24:*326–333.

Armstrong, W.D., Singer, L., Ensinck, J. and Rich, C.: 1964. Plasma fluoride concentrations of patients treated with sodium fluoride. *J. Clin. Invest., 43:*555.

Åslander, A.: 1961. Lifetime teeth. *N.Y. J. Dent., 10:*346–348.

Austen, K.F., Dworetzky, M., Farr, R.S., *et al.:* 1971. A statement on the question of allergy to fluoride as used in the fluoridation of community water supplies. *J. Allergy, 47:*347–348.

Berry, W.T.C.: 1958. A study of the incidence of mongolism in relation to the fluoride content of the water. *Am. J. Ment. Defic., 62:*634–636.

Berry, R.J. and Trillwood, W.: 1963. Sodium fluoride and cell growth. *Br. Med. J.,* Oct. 26, p. 1064.

Call, R.A., Greenwood, D.A., Le Cheminant, W.H., *et al.:* 1965. Histological and chemical studies in man on effects of fluoride. *Public Health Rep., 80:*529–538.

Carlson, J.R.: 1966. *Studies on the Metabolism of Sodium Fluoride. I. Plasma Fluoride in Relation to Dietary Fluoride in Dairy Cattle.* Ph.D. Thesis, Univ., of Wisconsin, Madison.

Cass, R.M., Croft, J.D., Jr., Perkins, P., *et al.:* 1966. New bone formation in osteoporosis following treatment with sodium fluoride. *Arch. Intern. Med., 118:*111–116.

Douglas, T.E.: 1956. Fluoride dentifrice and stomatitis. *Northwest Med., 56:*1037–1039.

Geall, M.G. and Beilin, L.J.: 1964. Sodium fluoride and optic neuritis. *Br. Med. J., 2:*355–356.

Linsman, J.F. and McMurray, C.A.: 1943. Fluoride osteosclerosis from drinking water. *Radiology, 40:*474–484.

Marier, J.R., Rose, D. and Boulet, M.: 1963. Accumulation of skeletal fluoride and its implications. *Arch. Environ. Health, 6:*664–671.

McCann, H.G. and Bullock, F.A.: 1957. The effect of fluoride ingestion on the composition and stability of mineralized tissues of the rat. *J. Dent. Res., 36:*391–398.

Medical Letter: 1969. Fluoridated water, hemodialysis and renal disease. Vol. 11, pp. 67–68.

Rapaport, I.: 1959. Nouvelles recherches sur le mongolisme. A propos du rôle pathogenique de fluor. *Bull. Acad. Natl. Med. (Paris), 143:*367–370.

Roholm, K.: 1937. The fog disaster in the Meuse Valley, 1930: A fluorine intoxication. *J. Ind. Hyg. Toxicol., 19:*126–137.

Sauerbrunn, B.J.L., Ryan, C.M. and Shaw, J.F.: 1965. Chronic fluoride intoxication with fluorotic radiculomyelopathy. *Ann. Intern. Med., 63:* 1074–1078.

Taves, D.R.: 1966. Normal human serum fluoride concentrations. *Nature, 211*:192–193.

Taves, D.R.: 1968. Evidence that there are two forms of fluoride in human serum. *Nature, 217*:1050–1051.

Taves, D.R.: 1970. New approach to the treatment of bone disease with fluoride. *Fed. Proc., 29*:1185–1187.

Taves, D.R., Terry, R., Smith, F.A. and Gardener, D.E.: 1965. Use of fluoridated water in long-term hemodialysis. *Arch. Intern. Med., 115*:167–172.

Taylor, A.: 1954. Sodium fluoride in the drinking water of mice. *Dent. Dig., 60*:170–172.

Taylor, A. and Taylor, N.C.: 1965. Effect of sodium fluoride on tumor growth. *Proc. Soc. Exp. Biol. Med., 119*:252–255.

Waldbott, G.L.: 1956. Incipient fluorine intoxication from drinking water. *Acta. Med. Scand., 156*:157–168.

Waldbott, G.L.: 1957. Tetanic convulsions precipitated by fluoridated drinking water. *Confin. Neurol., 17*:339–347.

Zipkin, I., McClure, F.J. and Lee, W.A.: 1960. Relation of the fluoride content of human bone to its chemical composition. *Arch. Oral Biol., 2*: 190–195.

AUTHOR INDEX

SUBJECT INDEX

LIST OF TABLES

LIST OF FIGURES